Sexy, Lean and Strong After 50!

How I went from *Fat, Depressed and Divorced* to the *Best Shape of My Life...and How YOU Can, Too!*

Deb Dutcher

Table of Contents

To everyone determined to be their best self –

Sexy, Lean and Strong –

no matter what life has thrown at you
or how old you are!

To Natalia –
Thank you for all
the encouragement
and support!
Love –
Deb Dutcher

Foreword

There has never been a higher state of emergency than the silent catastrophe we are living today. Our body's ability to deal with stress is frayed, our ability to stay lean and strong has weakened, our ability to think positively and stay focused has become fogged and blurred. We have become an over-burdened, emotionally stressed-out society. We eat for comfort and not for health.

There are two aspects to health and wellness--the foods we choose and the nutrients obtained. It is all about how well our mind, body and spirit are able to take the food we consume, digest it and nourish us as a whole. We are under such great challenges today in North America when it comes to understanding how to choose the right foods to fuel our body and our mind. Our soils are depleted and our conventional food-crops are weak and deficient. They are not producing the antioxidants we desperately need and our bodies are craving the nutrients we lack. We turn to highly-processed, artificially-colored foods whose pretty packages promise results, creating false hope it will quench our cravings and desires.

Through-out our lives we use food as the foundation for love, belonging, comfort and reassurance. We try to satiate our longings for something or someone we wish we had, or eat ourselves into a food-coma over some great sadness. The food industry knows how to tap into and suck in emotional eaters, and keep health-conscious shoppers hooked, with the right marketing. According to the Journal of Consumer Psychology, people with strong emotions experience higher levels of food cravings, salivation and eating intentions. According to the study there are three mediators that drive cravings: emotional memories, weak impulse control, and the intensity of pleasure anticipation.

The confectionary, beverage and food industries know that our body has the ability to take in food and categorize it for later use based not only on nutrient content but also on a reward and pleasure basis as well. The next time we are in a similar emotional state we will reach for a particular food based on past experiences.

When your body chemistry is balanced, you are balanced and your body is getting all the nutrients it needs. You will display emotions and behaviors that are in alignment with a healthy mind and body. You are better able to cope with stressful and emotional situations and attune to the positive outcome more readily.

We are only scratching the surface on how our brain and gut are interconnected. Globally, more than 350 million people of all ages are suffering from depression and it affects approximately 14.8 million American adults aged 18 and older in a given year. Women are more affected by depression, possibly as the result of the intricate messaging of hormones throughout their lifetime.

Hormones are special chemicals usually found in the glands of our endocrine system that release messengers directly into the blood and travel to the appropriate cells. Our cells then respond to the message. We require microscopic amounts of hormones each day and this delicately-balanced system requires the right nutrients to obtain them. If nutrients are lacking we end up with an unravelled communication system. Our cells and our hormones require the right nutrients from our food and are also affected by environmental factors, lifestyle and stress levels, as well as our outlook on life.

Look at the food consumed today. The SAD diet (Standard American Diet) contains genetically-altered foods, grown in pesticide-laden, nutrient-deficient soil, containing manipulated synthetic nutrients and chemical concoctions that numb the senses and keep us coming back for more. These foods are so highly processed that the finished products result in fillers, preservatives, additives and extracts devoid of the vitamins, minerals and fatty acids, antioxidants and probiotics we need on a daily basis to keep our body and mind healthy.

So, what can we do? Remember, we have the ultimate choice. We need to get back to real, unprocessed organic foods that are grown in the earth and animals that feed off grasses, nourished by the earth. This, along with good digestion and supplementation, will help us to nourish our body, brain and our soul. Vitamins and minerals, along with good fats, help normalize hormones and aid in supporting neurotransmitters. Neurotransmitters help transmit our thoughts and our reactions to others' behaviors. We require fatty acids on a daily basis as we do not make them on our own. They are called "essential fatty acids" (EFA's) for a reason; they are essential to our body. Our nerves, brain, and thoughts require fatty acids.

We now know from the mounting research that probiotics can help shape the integrity of our cells, hormones and our brain function. We need probiotics and fermented foods on a daily basis. We need quality foods and supplementation on a daily basis in order to run our body and mind properly and, to help us cope with our stressful lives and to deal with the emotional situations we encounter.

This is true of Deb Dutcher, author of Sexy, Lean and Strong After 50! Deb's health suffered along with her ability to cope with the incredible traumatic experiences she and her family endured. As Deb began to change her lifestyle along with her diet she began to see the connections in how she was able to better handle stress and the emotional roller-coaster of her life. Deb's healthier lifestyle helped her to recover from her losses, bravely step out on her own and reinvent herself and her life.

Deb was inspired to learn more as she grew healthier and stronger and this led her to further her education in nutrition. She came to Sanoviv Medical Institute, a holistic, state-of-the-art, fully-licensed hospital and health resort, to fully understand alternative therapies and the role of supplemental nutrition in helping bodies stay healthy and recover from degenerative diseases. As the past Director of Nutrition and Program Development at Sanoviv Medical Institute in Baja California Mexico and, as an international speaker, I have had the honor of teaching thousands the core concepts of nutrition, digestion and healing. Deb devoured the holistic teachings of Sanoviv and it was an honor to have such an astute student thirsty for more in my program.

Deb realized that her body is a biological energy and chemistry lab made up of neurons, cells and biological processes involved in creating, rejuvenating, repairing, firing energy and electrical impulses. In order for Deb to get off her Mad-Body Mountain she had to understand the deeper complexities of nutrition, supplementation, movement and psycho-spiritual connection. She learned that she had to have a strong mental attitude to help in her journey to sexy, lean and strong. Understanding how emotions, physical endurance and the spiritual connection are key to being able to get through any difficulties, allowing our body and mind to stay lean and strong, was critical to her growth and recovery.

It was such an honor to have been given the gift to glimpse into Deb's life through her book. We truly do not know another until we take the time to listen to their story. Deb's story is of trouble, turbulence, sorrow and yet, such an inspiration on her journey back to sound health. Deb has gone from depression, divorce and denial to a strong, sexy, lean mind and body and, as a result; a happy woman by honoring and nourishing all aspects of her mind, body and soul.

After applying what she learned at Sanoviv, Deb certified as a Health Coach through the Institute for Integrative Nutrition. Deb began educating those over-fifty as to how they too could experience the positive effects of good nutrition and supplementation so that they can better navigate the perils of their life's journey; stronger and leaner. Deb has become a beacon of hope for those over fifty who truly want to be sexy, lean and strong; mind and body, at any age!

Grab a tissue and get ready to cry. Cheer out loud and be energized as you learn how to get off the "Mad-Body Mountain" and tame the Bratty, Brainless Binger, Chatty, Chewy Cathy, Debbie Downer and the Mean, Midnight Muncher.

We all have our difficult painful pasts. We all have hopes, dreams and desires that sometimes do not turn or manifest into what we were hoping. This is not an excuse to give up. There are times when you feel as though you have no control. That is the time when you must realize you are the control. We all have choices. Even if the choice we make is not the right one, we can make another choice to make it right. We must learn to never give up.

Deb does a brilliant job defining what you need to do in order to take control of your life once again. As she says, you must not just jump off of the Mad-Body Mountain. You need to come down the mountain by addressing the Ten Steps and make sure to strengthen, repair and prepare for your descent.

We need to learn how to tune into our body and listen to what it is saying. When we are angry, sad, depressed or feeling low, this is our body communicating to us that something is out of balance. Instead of dealing with the root-cause, we reach for medications, food or alcohol to treat the symptoms or numb the brain.

We have come to this horrible misconception that if we are hormonal we need medication. If we are sad, blue or depressed we need medication. If we are fat, too thin or not just right there is a medication for that too. I promise you; never, ever…EVER will you have a deficiency of a medication. Now, could you have a deficiency of B vitamins, Co-enzyme Q10 and magnesium, causing you to feel drained and unfocused? You bet! Can you have a deficiency of essential fatty acids, causing inflammation and unbalanced hormones? Absolutely!

We have to start tuning in and understanding how our nutritional needs impact our moods, behaviors and our ability to cope. Deb is a prime example of how feeding her body the right nutrients allowed her to get off of her Mad-Body Mountain. Deb shows us how we can each get off our mountains, with a plan tailored to the individual. Deb provides concrete information about the factors of the Mad-Body Syndrome, and how to address each with a blend of care for the mind, body and spirit.

Epigenetics has proven that we are not governed by our genes, rather our nutrition and external environmental influences. We need to wake up and smell the nutrient rich coffee alternatives and start taking responsibility for our health.

Sure, we can all be dealt horrible experiences in our lives. Deb is a prime example of the beautiful story of struggle and triumph and all the bumps and roadblocks that went along with it. Throughout her incredible life story she honored her life's lesson in order to heal. Many of us have forgotten we too have the ability to change the situation we are in. Deb does an incredible job of reminding us of this very crucial key to wellness and health at any age. Deb has been completely transparent about her journey in the hopes of helping others to step up and take responsibility. She will hold your hand in this step-by-step detailed outline. The most incredible journey you will ever take is the journey of YOU!

When Deb reflects back on her connection to food choices and what she had to deal with emotionally, she realizes that perhaps things could have gone differently. As she so eloquently says, "…maybe I might have been able to calm down some of the issues in my body, get more sleep, control the food-cravings, and mood-swings. I would have been better able to handle my children's melt-downs due to their puberty and their own raging hormones. I believe I might still be married to my first husband and we would have worked things out."

Junk foods leads to junk thoughts and behaviors along with poor concentration, anger, grief, panic attacks, nervousness, unrest, feeling unloved, guilt, easily frustrated, non-deservingness, restlessness, worry, crying spells, depression, fear and phobias.

Whole foods from fruits, vegetables, nuts, seeds, whole grains, legumes and quality meat, fish and poultry leads to grounded positive thoughts and behaviors. These include feeling full of life, happiness, feeling loved, good decision-making, connected, healthy, energetic, calm, intimate, eager to learn, grounded, alive, balanced and loved. Most of all, good nutrition leaves us feeling and looking great, enjoying incredible energy, along with helping us to become sexy, lean and strong, at any age!

Whatever it is that you are dealing with I highly recommend trying Deb's recommendations. Go through the Ten Steps. When you are ready to take the next step Deb will be there to help you get off the Mad-Body Mountain back to sexy, lean and strong with concrete strategies. As Deb says, "Every day, every bite, every thought, is another opportunity to grow and re-craft your body--at any age." Especially for those over the age of fifty who may feel it is too late and that their battle to get down their mountain is fruitless.

Sexy, Lean and Strong After 50! will help you learn it is never too late!

Enjoy,

Karen Langston CN, CNP, RNCP, NNCP, LE, LM, SIT

Past Director of Nutrition and Program Development for Sanoviv Medical Institute, Author of Healthified Pantry, founder of the Healthy Gut Advisor Weekend Intensive.

Introduction

Good for you! You are determined to be sexy, lean and strong! I am 60+, and I am exactly that. But it wasn't always that way. I have been up in the obese range, down in the skinny range and, for 12+ years now I am right where I want to be – strong, lean and easily fitting into a Size 8. However, size is not the important thing – it is all about how you feel and your body being able to do whatever you want to. It is about being able to hike all day and dance all night! It is about sleeping like a baby and waking up to do something fun the next day! If you work, you want to be able to focus, be a high-performing business manager, owner or employee, and then exercise and play, long and hard, without feeling exhausted and depleted. But, can you?

Today, I look like I have it all and it is easy, yet I have had many problems to overcome – physical, emotional, life-crisis. Many of my clients have been through Hell and back, and I know exactly how they feel. There are several key stressors in life: Birth, Death, Marriage, Job Change or Loss, Move, Illness, Hospitalization, Divorce. Going through too many in one timeframe can create real stress in the body and trigger illness. I went through four of the eight in a period of eighteen months, including multiple moves. I know what happens when you are hit so many times you are not sure you can get back up, or even want to. I know the complete loss of energy or drive or desire to address your physical condition. I know the total sense of despair that drives one to want to just end it and leave this life. During that first Year of Loss, I would get up every day, knowing there was someone worse off that I was supposed to help. I would share my story, help them with their diet and get them on the supplements that were helping me. Being able to help gave me a reason to keep going. They would improve and send me more people to help.

Now, I want to help everyone I cannot meet in person. I want to share my process and learnings and help save someone from losing home or family or livelihood because they are chemically-imbalanced, over-fed, under-nourished, and depleted, as I was.

I am going to share with you my journey out of my tough years on top of Mad-Body Mountain to today. Today I am able to keep depression, arthritis, migraines, weight, hay-fever and skin problems at bay with a combination of healthy eating, good supplements, bi-weekly chiropractic care, daily exercise and safe, gentle and pure skin-care. I have not had an operation or been hospitalized. I am not on any prescriptions. I have not had flus or colds for more than five years, nor a flu shot! I am overflowing with energy and happiness!

I tell everyone, "No matter how bad it is, you can have some improvement. It is never too late to take back your health." I have clients in their 50s and 60s who are running marathons, competing in triathlons and swimming Alcatraz. They are the extreme. I like to hike, bike, jog, dance, swim and climb hills. You may just want to have enough energy to play with your kids and grandkids, or, reduce dependence on medication. It all starts with taking inventory – of your lifestyle, your habits, thoughts and desires. What are you looking for? Energy Sabotagers! And then you are going to eliminate them, one-by-one and develop healthy habits that will last for a lifetime.

Deb Dutcher, Health Coach
Brentwood, California

Prologue – The Storms Hit

There I was, sitting in my cubicle, poring over the documents for the system cutover. I was the Global Project Manager for a high-tech firm in Silicon Valley, working at a project to bring in a new corporate software system. I had been married to my college sweetheart for nineteen years. I was becoming a first-time mom of two children at the age of forty. The years had been blissful – we were DINKs – Double Income No Kids. We were both earning six figures and the only creature we had to worry about was our cat. My husband was the most understanding, patient and loving man on the planet! I was madly in love still.

As we were not able to have children, we had been looking at adoption. In 1992, we became foster parents and waited for a placement. Our children came to live with us on Valentine's Day of 1993. We adopted them May of 1994. They were a "sibling-group" – a boy and girl, half-brother and sister. Same mom, different dads. The mom was Caucasian and the dads were Mexican. Our son never met his father as his mother had become pregnant while a teen-aged runaway in Mexico, then returned to the States to give birth. Both children were born in Northern California. Our daughter's birth-father terminated his parental rights while the birth-mom was in prison. Both children had been through abuse and had some real issues. They had been in foster care for eighteen months and it was time for a final placement.

Social Services explained that they only knew a portion of what the children had been through, but it included emotional and physical abuse for the boy and sexual abuse for the girl. They told us that the real behavior problems would hit when the kids hit puberty. We were so naïve! It did not stop us as we had fallen in love with the children from our first meeting. At that time, she was five, turning six and he was eight, turning nine. Both were love-starved and beautiful!

Their birth-mom was in prison, with parental rights being terminated.

The birth-grand-mother was an alcoholic and had turned-down caring for Abe. Raquele's birth-father had been determined unfit. The children were told they had no permanent home on Thanksgiving, 1992. We met them early December, and they were placed with us just two months after we met them, in February of 1993, instead of the six months we had been promised. There was no real "getting to know you" time. They moved in on Valentine's Day, 1993, and all hell broke loose!

We were dealing with behavior issues from two children, born drugs-in-utero, who both had ADD and pre-disposition to chemical substance abuse. There was acting-out at school, and temper tantrums at home. Both would refuse to do simple chores or even brush their hair or teeth. We were looking for solutions to handling all the anger.

Originally, the children had therapists who were provided by Social Services. Abe's was being ruled by Abe, who would lay upside-down in a chair in the man's office, telling him all sorts of lies about his sexual activity, at the age of nine! I sat in on two of these "free sessions" and determined that they were worthless and that we needed someone who could really see past all the bluff to the real child in pain. Meantime, Raquele was being seen by another therapist who was working with her on the sexual abuse. We were definitely in over our heads!

The years in elementary and middle school for both children were frantic, to say the least. By 1999, our son was 14 and his sister was 11, and neither wanted to be parented. We were seeing three therapists – hers, his and ours. My husband was gone for weeks at a time. My parenting skills were lacking and I did not control my temper well.

My parents were divorced when I was nine and, by age eleven, I was often left to care for my three younger siblings, without much of a role-model. Force and yelling were my two tactics for maintaining order. This does not work well when your own children are also prone to yelling and force. Plus, when a child has lived through abuse, yelling and force are useless. But, they were my primary parenting tools. That, and blackmail and bribery. Basically I was operating as a teen-aged mom, the way I had with my brothers and sisters when left to care for them. I had no skills and did not even know what I was doing wrong.

Upon his return, my husband would play the mediator, counseling each of us and trying to restore order. Unfortunately, he traveled a lot, for weeks at a time, and much of the time the children and I were careening around the home in emotional upheaval. He would come home, all the sins would be trotted-out, the complaints lodged, the plans put in place, and then off he would go and it would get out-of-control again.

Add to that the stresses of two high-tech careers, long commutes and late hours, and you can imagine the toll it took on both of us and the marriage.

Abe's Story

My son was so smart and really knew how to work the system. He asked us, after they were living with us for a few months, "Why haven't we been permanently placed? It is supposed to happen within eighteen months of being in the system and we are still foster children." His main goals were to turn eighteen and 1) sue the abusive foster father and 2) go to Mexico to find his birth-dad. The dinner conversation would revolve around all the abuse that had been done to him and his sister. He had tried to protect her, but he was seven and she was four. Ultimately, at age seven, he called his Social Services worker and got them out of that home. No charges were ever filed, because there was no proof. But other children who came from that home to another he was sent to told the same type of stories of abuse. It broke our hearts!

Before the birth-mom's parental rights were terminated, before the adoption was final, we facilitated visits with the birth-mom. On one visit, Abe asked his mom if she was planning to have any more children. She said, "No, they tied my tubes in the prison and I can't have any more kids." He told her, "Good, 'cuz you are a lousy mom."

At the age of four, she would leave him alone to care for Raquele, then one year old and in diapers, with one dollar for food all day, while she was off doing drugs and entertaining johns. He would cross a busy highway to beg from the only store near-by, a See's candy store. At the age of 8, all his baby-teeth were abcessed. Abe never asked for candy, just asparagus, artichokes, broccoli and fresh fruit.

By the time he reached fourteen, he was out-of-control. His grades went from 3.2 in 8th grade to .2 his freshman year in high school. We were constantly dealing with police coming to the home, then Juvenile Hall and Juvenile Court. Neither of us had any experience with "The System" and were clueless. My husband had to miss a court-date due to his business travels and when I explained his absence to the judge, I was told that he had to be there and there was no excuse! It took hours to have a case heard and you had to sit in a room with all kinds of scary people, there for their children. We were totally out of our comfort zone. My son's case-worker had 120 kids to deal with and, since he was non-violent, he was not a high-priority.

We tried to use medication to help him. We had him evaluated at the Amen Clinic, with resting and active brain-scan MRIs. The results were extremely dis-heartening. According to the findings, Abe had sections of his brain missing – anger management, impulse control and ability to understand consequences. Yet he was borderline brilliant in terms of intelligence. According to the doctors, he was basically a socio-path. That seemed to explain the lying, stealing and drug-use. We tried a medication cocktail and it appeared to help. But, by high-school he was refusing the medication. And his therapist, herself a former run-away and drug-user, advised us not to force him.

Abe had tremendous leadership skills. He ran with a pack of kids and could get them to do whatever he wanted. I joked with my husband that he was perfect for a con-man or politician. He also had a "Golden Heart", evidenced by the care he gave to babies and older, infirm people. But, there was very little conscience and no concept of right and wrong. He got out of Juvenile Hall, went off for a 4th of July celebration and next thing we knew a policeman was at the door, saying he had just been caught shoplifting a bottle of Jack Daniels.

In California, at age 16, the child must tell the judge what they want. Abe wanted to go to a three-week survival camp in Utah to see if it would help him. He was cutting school, drinking and doing grass and possibly other drugs. We never got the full story. Ultimately I used stock-option money to have him sent to a camp in Utah. Once done with the camp, we went to Utah to bring him home and he said he could not come back to the Bay Area as there were too many temptations.

We found a co-ed therapeutic high-school in Utah and placed him there. He drove them crazy, hitting on the girls and, when put in solitary just sleeping through it or writing angry poetry. His behavior never changed. The male school director (a former prison psychiatrist) literally called us crying after a few months of this and asked to have him removed. We had a survival camp group from Idaho come get him without telling him, for the shock value, and, for three weeks, he lived outside in the snow, logging, sleeping in a teepee and going on a trek over an ice bridge in Canada. He loved it! When he "graduated" he asked again not to be brought home. We found another school, again in Utah, and moved him in there.

Through the therapy at that school, they found out he had been deep into drugs and fight-clubs back in California. By then, he was seventeen and wanted to get into the Marines. To do that he had to go off his meds. That meant he could not stay at the school.

By this time, 2000, I had become a VP at a start-up and an overnight Internet millionaire. I cashed out enough stock to put down on a 75-acre ranch in Placerville. The rancher next to me ran his cattle on my land so, when Abe left his school, I asked if Abe could bunk in there. I paid room and board and gave the rancher extra money for Abe for his spending-money. We moved him in, got him into the high school, and went home to deal with the next storm – our daughter and her issues with alcohol, drugs and men.

Raquele's Story

Raquele wanted nothing more than to have love from her brother. In the beginning, when they first moved in, he would push her away as he harbored resentment because he felt she had had preferential treatment at the third foster home. One day, nine months after they moved in, he actually hugged her good-night and told her he loved her. My husband and I both got tears in our eyes, looked at each other and said, "That is why we did this." It was one of the happier times.

As a child of six, Raquele exhibited some disturbing behaviors. She would slip her sweater provocatively off her shoulders and pout and act really sexy. I would have long conversations about appropriate behavior when she had boyfriends and answer questions about what was the right way to act with men. Of course, it went right over her head and had no real impact, based on what went on in her teens.

My daughter was extremely resistant to any sort of parenting. Our first year she told me I was the "worst mom she had ever had!" She was five and I had asked her to pick up her toys. She had had four moms before me – neglectful birth-mom, an emergency home for a few weeks, the seven-month placement with her brother where they were both allegedly abused, and then separate, therapeutic foster homes. After which, eighteen months into the system, they were placed with us.

When she said that to me, it really hurt. Especially since I knew one mom was a drug-using prostitute and another had been abusive. Yet, all the yelling did not deter me from expecting certain actions – do your homework, keep yourself neat and tidy and pick-up your room. So began our War-of-Wills in the first year. The War-of-Wills continued throughout her teen years.

By the time she was thirteen, her brother was out of the home. We were dealing with all her anger and distaste for authority. We would ask her to do something, she would say yes, but never do it. Homework was finished but rarely turned in. At 14, she started sneaking out of the house and hooking up with older men. She ran away while my mom was staying there when we left for a trip. She got kicked out of two high-schools and ended up in a Continuation school. She tried to commit suicide, swallowing a bottle of Tylenol when told she could not see her birth-mom for Mother's Day. I spent that Mother's Day by her bed in the hospital, after they pumped her stomach and put her on suicide watch.

Finally, I quit my six-figure engineering vice-president position to stay home with her to see if we could get things under control. This totally back-fired as she had been hosting parties at the home on her half-days, which apparently included drinking and possibly, sex. Now she could not blow-off steam and all hell broke loose.

We fought all the time. She yelled horrible things at me and I fought back like a teenager. My husband went on anti-depressants, I was going through menopause and also on anti-depressants and Raquele was going through puberty and on ADD meds.

While she was on her fourth stay at Juvenile Hall, a twenty-eight day stint this time, my husband went to a parenting conference the Saturday before she was due back and came home to say we had to implement rules and a contract. I was relieved, as I had been suggesting that for years. I had even successfully put together contracts with the kids while he was gone, but he would reverse them on his return.

I said, "Great, let's get it figured out now." He said, "Not tonight." I pushed and he finally told me I could not stay in the home when she came back, that she had told him she could not live with me. I was driving her crazy. He told me, "You are the adult and can take care of yourself. She is a child and I have to take care of her." He said it would kill him if he had to see us fight again. He would have a heart attack. He said we needed to separate for six months till he could get things under control, without me in the home. My heart broke. I told him I did not want him to die and that I knew she and I would fight

18

again. I agreed I had to leave the home. We cried and held each other all night.

Deb's Story

After that night, we lived like strangers in our home, until I could move out. After twenty-nine years of a loving marriage, he cut me off. No hugs, no sweet talks, no kisses. He moved into the guest room off the kitchen. When I would try to hug him, he turned to stone and I would tremble head-to-toe, hanging onto his neck.

He would not agree to any more counseling for the two of us. He said I had had all the chances and I never changed. He had to focus on saving Raquele. He could not lose another child. He felt he had lost Abe to his demons and he could not lose her.

I could not bear it. He had been the anchor of my life – a perfect, loving partner – my best friend, confidante, supporter, lover, husband. I was completely empty without him. One night I was so distraught, I gathered all the clothing and gifts he had given me, piled them on my Oriental carpet and sat there with the scissors pointed at my stomach. He caught me as I was contemplating how to just stop living by committing hara-kiri and shook me out of it.

I moved out for a time to the ranch and then to a friend's. I came back for some counseling in the home which was for Raquele and for potential reconciliation.   Raquele would have none of it, clamming up and refusing to answer the therapist's questions or engage in any dialogue with me.

I tried two more times to end it – standing in the dark in the street in front of a moving car, and planning to drive off a cliff -- and chickened-out each time.

It took a while for it to sink in. He and I would have to part. I could not stay in the home and it would have to be sold. All my money was in our home, the ranch and supporting Abe. My internet stock had become worthless, so all I had was my savings. It was dwindling fast with the mortgage on the ranch. I had no income.

I moved into an apartment a few blocks away. My furniture was a futon, a dresser and a kitchen counter stool. My TV rested on a large packing box, covered with a tablecloth. Everything else was at the family home to get it ready to sell. My husband had to co-sign for me on the apartment as I had no credit in my own name. I would go back and forth to the ranch and try to maintain it alone.

At the ranch, when I could not sleep, I spent hours crying on the floor, curled around my beautiful, loving Black Lab, Boomer. I would write in my journal and wonder how I was going to survive.

How Menopause Affected the Prior Events

I went through menopause from 1989 to 1999. It was very early, as I was thirty-seven when it started, right about the time we were trying to get pregnant. A fertility doctor put me on a fertility-drug, Clomid, double-dose. I ended up in three fender-benders as I would become dis-oriented behind the wheel. I would think I was stepping on the gas or brake and it would be the opposite. I was rear-ending people or they were rear-ending me. I took myself off the meds and we decided to adopt.

During the peri-menopause and menopause, I did not sleep, I put on weight, I had mood-swings and cried all the time. That is, when I wasn't screaming and raging at the world, but especially my new role as a mom of two very troubled and difficult children. I had horrible hot flashes, day and night. I had migraines that began at 4 p.m. and went on till 2 a.m., during which time I could not be in the light or have any food. I would lay on the floor with an ice-pack on my forehead and just try to endure. My temple would throb, my eye would stream and my jaw would hurt. If I took anything for the pain, I would throw it up. I had no energy and did not manage stress well. I did not know anything about nutrition. I was eating a Snickers bar for a pick-me-up at 3 p.m. and suffering with a migraine one hour later. I drank very little water. I did not know anything about hormonal fluctuation and the effects on the emotions.

My therapist put me on Zoloft. It did not help. I did not realize that much of my rage and inability to control my temper was due to the raging chemical and hormonal storm going on inside me, sensitivity to sugar and need for more water.

Today, I feel that, had I been able to calm down some of the issues in my body, get more sleep, control the food-cravings, and mood-swings, I would have been better able to handle my children's melt-downs due to their puberty and their own raging hormones. I believe I might still be married to my first husband and we would have worked things out.

The vitamins, dietary changes, and nutritional supplements I put my menopausal clients on now are making a huge difference in their stress levels, sleeping, weight loss and reducing the hot-flashes. I believe they are necessary to get safely through the hormonal fluctuations and retain sanity. Men have a similar issue as their testosterone starts fluctuating. Our family dynamic was definitely adversely impacted by my and my husband's "mid-life crises", triggered by hormones and aging, at the same time as our children's puberty and emotional issues.

The most important thing to me now is to help others to normalize the body's cravings, addictions, hormonal surges, emotional swings and get them back to a "happy body" state and off Mad-Body Mountain. This will ultimately allow their relationships to be smoother and easier to manage successfully.

The driving reasons I now am a Health Coach and started Abe's Heart of Gold Foundation to work with youth-at-risk are:

- I want to save other families from going through what mine went through--emotional upheaval, stress and loss
- I want to help women struggling with the horrific chemical changes that occur in menopause--weight gain, mood swings, lack-of-energy and sex-drive
- I want to help the men struggling with the aging process and stubborn fat around the mid-section, lack of energy and sex-drive
- I want to save kids from self-medicating with drugs and alcohol
- I want to help everyone understand sugar is as much of a drug as cocaine
- I want to sound a call to everyone who is over-medicating with prescription drugs, getting fatter and feeling worse daily, that there is another way.

Chapter 1 –
Overview of Mad-Body Mountain;
How Mad Is Your Body?

What is "Mad-Body Mountain"?

My term for what happens to our bodies when we have put ourselves last for too long – working at a career, being a parent, running a home, becoming a caregiver. One day we look down at a shapeless blob, with health issues, and wonder, "How did I get here?" I compare it to having started on a hike and, much later, found yourself on top of a mountain, not sure how to get off. You are staring down at a steep cliff, and have no idea how to get down.

Get me off *Mad-Body Mountain!*

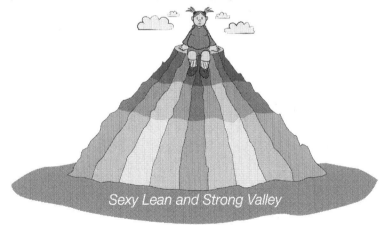

Sexy Lean and Strong Valley

Many of my clients have been through divorce, lost a home, spouse, parent, even lost a child. Some have lost jobs or businesses. They are dealing with bodies that have been ignored and are in crisis. I am able to share with them my own struggles and losses and show them that there is hope. It just takes focusing on what will help your body the most.

Every day, every bite, every thought, is another opportunity to grow and re-craft your body. Even those with disabilities and injuries can work to improve. The key is you cannot just jump back to the valley floor. To get off Mad-Body Mountain back to Sexy, Lean and Strong Valley, you have to have a plan and a trail-map and do it in stages. I did not really understand that back during my storms, and it took a while to acknowledge what I was going through, accept that I had to make a change and then, implement it. Plus, on the way down the mountain, you have to stop, evaluate what is happening, what you want to happen next, and adjust the plan to get to the next goal.

So, as you join me in my journey down my "mad-body mountain", I will share you with what I have learned about the best ways down and how to stay off.

It is not really that hard, and yet is perhaps the hardest thing you will do – taking back your health and mental well-being. And yes, there are some key nutritional changes, including vitamins and supplements, without which it would have been much harder and time-consuming for me. You can get healthy on organic foods and exercise, but, if you are struggling with anything, you may need more. For me, I choose safe supplements (my term for it is: radical nutritional intervention), with no side-effects, over the medication I used to be on. Modern medicine did not keep me off the "Mad-Body Mountain". It actually helped put me there. It puts most of my clients there.

At the end of the journey/book you will have been able to find out what is going to help your body release fat, permanently, and create the Sexy, Lean and Strong body you want. You are going to greet every day with the knowledge you can accomplish anything you want to. You will know how to reduce or eliminate medication (after your doctor agrees) and how to calm yourself and get through the tough days and nights. I am going to share all the things that helped me, and give you all the shortcuts to help you be Sexier, Leaner and Stronger!

So Jump In and Let's Do This!

Here are some key concepts we need to go over:

- Bodies get mad when they are not fed right, hydrated, exercised right or given enough sleep
- Bodies get really mad when they are depleted of the essential proteins, enzymes, hormones, vitamins, minerals and antioxidants they need to do their repairs and rebuilding over an extended period
- Without all the building-blocks and enough sleep for the repair cycles, the body degenerates and ages, prematurely
- You are responsible for the condition of your body – not your parents, heritage, race, cultural mores, spouse, kids, friends or your physician
- If you want to get Sexy, Lean and Strong, it will take focus and commitment, but you can do it!
- There is a Ten Step process to getting off the Mountain, and, without addressing these steps, you are just jumping off with no parachute!

Ten Steps to Get Off Mad-Body Mountain

1. Identify your Stage on the Mountain
2. Decide: Do You Need to Strengthen, Repair and Prepare for Your Descent?
3. How to Strengthen, Repair and Prepare for Your Descent: Fix the Top 3 to 5 Worst Habits
4. Discover Your Optimal Nutrition Strategy
5. Design Your Best Exercise Program
6. Develop Your Self-Care and Stress-Management Strategy
7. Make Your Relationships Work for You
8. Strap on Your Pack and Let's Hike!
9. Stay on the Path; Adjust as Needed
10. Celebrate your Arrival to Sexy, Lean and Strong Valley!

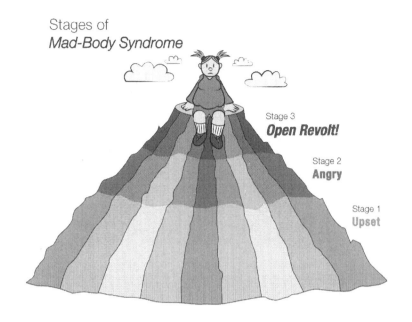

Stages of
Mad-Body Syndrome

Stage 3
Open Revolt!

Stage 2
Angry

Stage 1
Upset

Step 1: Identify Your Stage On The Mountain

In order to determine where you are on the mountain and how long it will take to get down, you have to determine what stage you are in Mad-Body Syndrome. Here are the stages I have defined:

Stage 1 – Upset

Stage 2 – Angry

Stage 3 – Open Revolt

Three Stages of the Mad-Body

Stage 1: Upset – 5 to 20 lbs overweight

Description: Uncomfortable, gassy, farting, mild or infrequent headaches, low energy, some trouble sleeping, sinus problems, sporadic exercise, a bit depressed

Avg. Descent Time: 30 – 45 days to lose up to 12 pounds and feel much better; another 30 to 45 days to lose another 8 to 12 pounds and feel amazing

Stage 2: Angry – 25 to 40 lbs overweight

Description: Digestive disorders, bowel disorders, frequent headaches, sinus problems, big problems sleeping, very low energy, mild to moderate joint pain, lower back pain, food allergies; on one or more meds to control issues; pre-diabetic

Avg. Descent Time: 60 to 90 days to lose up to 25 lbs and feel better; another 60 to 90 days to lose another 10 – 15 lbs and feel great!

May require a Strengthen, Repair and Prepare phase, usually one to two weeks.

Stage 3: Open Revolt – 40+ lbs overweight

Description: Major digestive issues – bloating after meals, severe aches and pains; may be diagnosed with arthritis, diabetes, high cholesterol, high blood pressure, auto-immune disease or cancer; on multiple medications

Avg. Descent Time: Usually requires a Strengthen, Repair and Prepare phase to correct Top 3 to 5 worst habits, add in some supplements, get some sleep and prepare for the descent. SRP may last one to two months until body and spirit are ready for full overhaul. Apply Stage 2 estimates for weight loss after SRP.

To help you understand these stages, and identify where you currently are, I am going to use some client case-studies. I am not using their real names as I don't want to break client-coach confidentiality. Note that you can be between stages as well.

Stage 1: Upset

About one-third of my coaching practice is working with Stage 1 – Upset folks – they are usually in their mid-30s to late-40s.

Something health-wise is worrying them, or they just have to go to an event and nothing fits, or they are just tired of being tired. They are at the easiest stage and we can usually get some great results in the first 45 to 60 days. Here is a typical couple who were in Stage 1.

Sandy and John are an adorable couple in their mid-30s, one a teacher and one a school psychologist. They have two sweet children, a four-year old and a one-year old. Both found themselves worn-out and carrying twenty-plus extra pounds that would not come off.

The solution was getting them on the right nutritional program, including a jump-start cleanse to kick the sugar cravings, plus the right supplements to bring up their energy and help them sleep. This ultimately gave them both the energy to exercise, plan and make healthy meals and release the extra weight.

John lost 18 lbs and 11 inches in 60 days, and Sandy lost 13 lbs and 9 inches in 75 days. Sandy went through three weeks of SRP before jumping to the Jumpstart 5-day cleanse. John went straight to the 5-day cleanse and then to the Transform phase.

Both got off Mad-Body Mountain just in time for their vacation to Kauai. Sandy got into a bikini for the first time in years!

Stage 2: Angry

Another third of my coaching practice is working with the Stage 2 - Angry heading to Stage 3 – Open Revolt. These are successful executives, entrepreneurs and harried parents, most in their 40s and 50s, who have been alerted to things needing to change by new aches and complaints, unexplained and stubborn weight-gain, or a parent's decline. They are worried they are going to end up sick or on medication and stay fat forever.

Marnie, 54, came to me frustrated over her inability to lose weight and dealing with an increasing number of food allergies. Her skin itched, she was restless, waking up between 11 p.m. and 1 a.m., and she was not getting to the gym. She had put on thirty pounds and it would not budge, despite eating mostly salads and lean proteins. She quit her four-day-a-week spinning class because the scale would not budge!

By delving into her family and personal health history, I realized she was dealing with a toxic liver. When asked, she revealed not only her mother but sister had the same type of food allergies and skin issues. Her mother had passed away several years prior, having first been hospitalized with liver problems.

We needed to do more than a jump-start cleanse. We needed to find out what was triggering the imbalance and reverse it. Marnie already could not eat strawberries, almonds, shellfish, dairy or gluten. But, we needed to go deeper.

The liver is the soldier of the body, it has to process all medicine, toxins and chemicals before it can process food. A bulging tummy and food allergies will often signify a liver imbalance. For Marnie, I added probiotics, daily multi-vitamin and minerals, plus a liver support product with milk-thistle, alpha-lipoic acid, turmeric and Vitamin C. I also used the teachings in The Liver Cleansing Diet by Dr. Sandra Cabot (see References). This is an eight-week program, designed to get the liver de-toxed and functioning optimally again.

She also increased her water intake. Optimal water intake should be at least one-half of your body weight.

By the end of the first three weeks, Marnie was sleeping through the night, the itchy skin was subsiding and she was feeling very energetic.

She went back to the gym, began a cardio and toning regimen, and, at the end of the eight weeks, we started on a weight-loss program, using a cleanse and then continuing on the maintain liver health diet.

That program created a nine-pound weight loss in just three weeks, once the liver cleanse was over.

Stage 3: Open Revolt

Then there are the clients who are on top of the mountain, way up in Stage 3 – Open Revolt. They are usually in their 50s and 60s, or even older. Many have been diagnosed with an illness – diabetes, obesity, fibromyalgia, arthritis, heart problems, hypothyroid, high cholesterol, high blood-pressure and worse. They are on multiple medications, their weight is out-of-control and they have absolutely no energy. They know they are making poor choices but feel powerless to stop and don't know where to start. Often their decline has been triggered by a life-crisis: long-term stress, loss of a job, home or loved-one. They are despondent and feel they cannot get off the Mad-Body Mountain. Food is their comfort and nemesis.

Julie, then 62, came to me in May, after losing her husband five months earlier, just a few days before Christmas. She had been caring for him for over four years. He was twenty years her senior and had been dealing with heart problems. She went upstairs to do some Christmas cards, came down and he had passed-away of a massive heart attack.

They had run their real-estate business together for over twenty years. She tried to keep everything going, along with dealing with all the family issues.

By the time she came to me she was carrying sixty extra pounds on a 5'4" frame, weighing-in at 196 lbs. She had no energy and was on multiple medications – high blood-pressure, heart medication and joint medication. She had so much pain in her back that she was bowed-over. Her knees hurt constantly.

The first thing we had to address was her lack of sleep, not eating enough good food, having no energy and being on several medications. It is not easy to lose weight when the liver is processing medication all the time, so the first thing was to do a SRP cycle to get her sleeping better and having more energy. She began to start the day with a healthy breakfast, and added some supplements to support her liver, heart and a healthy blood pressure.

The Strengthen, Repair and Prepare phase lasted one week. Followed with the jump-start 5-day cleanse, and then the full Transform program. Nine months later she is a svelte 138 pounds, dating and full of energy! And her doctor has her off all her medications.

Now, What About You?

Ask yourself, what Level of Mad is your body? You can be between stages – there is a 1.5, 2.5 and 3.5 (where you are literally falling off the back of the mountain). They all require you to do the same things. Stop the habits, thoughts and food-choices that are making your body Mad!!!

The goal is to get off the mountain and back to pre-Stage 1 – Stage 0 – Sexy, Lean and Strong Valley. This is where there are no real health complaints, you are at a comfortable weight and it is easy to maintain. You can do any reasonable activity, whenever you feel like it – bike, hike, run, play sports, exercise, work all night, dance for hours. Anything you want or need to do. And you will not crash or collapse afterwards, or be in excruciating pain. You will have arrived at Sexy, Lean and Strong Valley, and you never have to leave.

Word of caution: Do not attempt to wrench yourself down the mountain with crash diets or hours of daily exercise! You are not ready. Once you have determined which stage you are in, please move cautiously and determinedly, but not hastily. Realize that you may have to pause at each level as you descend. This journey is much like a strenuous hike up or down a mountain. You pause a third of the way up and again two-thirds of the way up, as well as on the return.

You do this because you need to check-in on your body, to see how it is reacting to a new program, where you are getting feedback and what kind of feedback. You may plateau for a while. The weight does not always come off week-after-week. There are adjustment cycles, and then you need to evaluate if you need to amp-up or switch-up the exercise and the nutrition.

We don't want to drop tons of weight too fast. For one thing, as we are older our bodies don't snap-back and we will get droopy-skin. One to two pounds a week is what to target. You can release more, but you need to make sure you are adequately nourished, not faint or feeling weak.

Once you have determined which mad-body stage you are in, then you can begin to plan your descent off the mountain. If you are in late Stage 2 or full Stage 3, a preparatory phase I call Strengthen, Repair and Prepare will be necessary. This is the phase where you have to be really good to yourself. Usually your body is quite depleted – you are not sleeping and you have no energy. You are using caffeine and sugar to keep going. Sometimes you are dealing with emotional blocks.

For most it takes a minimum of one to two weeks preparing the body – increasing energy and stamina and sleeping better. Adding supplements if necessary. Cleaning up the eating habits and bringing in some walking does wonders. Often we can lose weight in this phase, but the goal is to just start feeling better. Journaling on food, emotions, sleep and exercise will help you recognize what is out-of-balance.

Just like Julie, my Stage 3 client, you cannot just start down the mountain and onto the right habits. Your brain will not cope. My client is a good example. She wanted to lose weight but it was clear she was stuck in a desperate place emotionally. She had not gone through the grieving process, which meant that before I could put her through a real lifestyle change, I had to get her body stronger and capable of dealing with the deprivations of dumping the junk-foods and bringing in the healthy ones, while tackling her emotional state.

As part of Julie's program, we did some grief-release and she joined a grief-support group. This allowed her to open up to others who had experienced a loss, to share her anguish in a safe, supportive environment, which then made it possible for her to manage the new lifestyle.

If you are in a bad state – forty-plus pounds overweight, or on meds, post-surgery or chemo, or just totally run-down and exhausted, your body may not be ready for that diet or cleanse you have been considering. Too many people jump into a diet or cleanse or try fasting, hoping to drop some weight, and actually aggravate their problems.

There is something called the "starvation response" – this is when your body thinks it is not going to get enough food, slows down the metabolism and stores fat in the fat cells , particularly the mid-section. All because the body is still a Stone Age creature and, when it is stressed, it wants to be able to handle anything – famine, running from a big predator, whatever. If you are stressed and dealing with a Mad Body, then it will be very hard to lose weight. You will have to calm down your body and increase your nutrition before you can implement major changes.

Several of my clients have dealt with this phenomenon. One, Jane, a nurse of 53, had been through gastric-bypass surgery, lost over 100 pounds, then eaten her way back to an extra 45 pounds. She was eating too little, at the wrong times for her schedule--38 hour graveyard shifts and 4 hour round-trip commutes. By moving her to four meal-replacements shakes, and a light meal, during her 38-hour shift, she dropped 15 lbs in two months. She is continuing to lose gradually, week by week.

Gastric-bypass surgery is one way to drop weight when all else fails. The problem that I see with my clients who have had it is, they lose stomach capacity but then sometimes they eat and stretch it right back out. Then, they are really frustrated. The other problem is they have to eat enough protein, in easily-absorbed forms, to stay well-nutriented. Most of my gastric-bypass clients do really well on protein and fiber shakes, along with the supplements, due to the ease of digestion and metabolization.

Chapter 2 – Do You Need to Strengthen, Repair and Prepare?

In Chapter 1 you found out you are on the Mad-Body Mountain and you need to get down. You figured out what stage you are. If you are confused, please contact me through: www.sexyleanandstrong.com and I will help.

Step 2: Decide – Do You Need to Strengthen, Repair And Prepare?

The most important decision is whether you are going to need to do the Strengthen, Repair and Prepare phase before tackling the climb down. This is similar to training for a mountain climb or athletic endeavor. We have to make sure your body and brain is ready to take on dietary changes, new exercises and habits.

Before you determine whether you are going to go through SRP, you need to review the Factors of the Mad-Body to determine how mad your body is. If you have a really mad body, you will need to use "baby-steps" as your body needs to overcome its issues gradually, not all at once. Just as you cannot quit your meds cold-turkey, you cannot jump down to the valley from the top of your mountain. That is why I use the prep-phase, Strengthen, Repair and Prepare. We have to get the body strong enough to deal with the changes, and not try to just jump-off of the mountain!

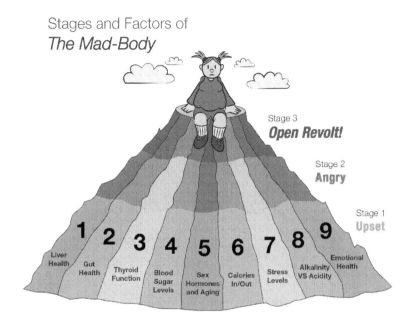

Stages and Factors of
The Mad-Body

Stage 3
Open Revolt!

Stage 2
Angry

Stage 1
Upset

1 Liver Health
2 Gut Health
3 Thyroid Function
4 Blood Sugar Levels
5 Sex Hormones and Aging
6 Calories In/Out
7 Stress Levels
8 Alkalinity VS Acidity
9 Emotional Health

Stages and Factors of the Mad-Body

First, the sections are numbered in terms of importance (per my findings).

1. The Liver has to be functioning in optimal condition to keep the rest of the body clean and detoxed.

2. The Gut has to be able to extract the nutrition and deliver it to the body.

3. The Thyroid needs to be balanced for the metabolism to be at the right levels.

4. Insulin has to stay level or you get blood-sugar spikes which can lead to metabolic syndrome and then, diabetes.

5. Aging and the amount of sex hormones will affect other areas of the body – emotions, cravings, metabolism, even the thyroid.

6. Calories in and calories out are important – too many calories with too little exercise and we gain weight. Too few and too much exercise and we get weak and can lose muscle. Even more important is the type of calories and how nutritious they are.

7. Stress is huge and we must have it under control to have balance and be able to function.

8. Alkalinity is driven by the amount of processed foods and animal protein vs raw vegetables, plant proteins and unprocessed foods.

9. Emotions control everything. Too much anger, sadness, fear will drive different hormones which will drive our desire, or lack of, to eat and exercise and, ultimately, affect our overall health.

If too many of these factors are off-track, then it will be very hard to get down the mountain. Determining which are most important for you is the entire point of Strengthen, Repair and Prepare. Just because I have listed certain factors last does not mean you may not need to address them first to get results. Remember the client who had to deal with grieving before anything else? It is almost impossible to make real progress getting down the mountain if you are suppressing your emotions and trying to just keep going.

Ask yourself:

- Am I getting 7 to 8 hours of sleep nightly? If not, why not?
- Do I drink at least half my weight in ounces of water a day?
- Do I have energy all day long? When do I slump?
- Can I walk away from salty or sugar-y foods, or comfort foods?
- Do I get at least 30 minutes of movement/exercise daily?
- Do I get my nine cups of vegetables daily?

If you have more than three that are No answers, you should do some period of SRP. My rule-of-thumb is work on three key points for two weeks and, once you correct them, then the rest. Once you can manage these habits, then you can add the harder changes that will be necessary to get you off the mountain.

Understanding who you are, what you are dealing with, and then, deciding to take it on is the most important step for Strengthen, Repair and Prepare. This is where you may need to get some help. Once you know *your* Top 3 to 5 areas to address, you start the actual Strengthen, Repair and Prepare process – Step 3.

If you are having trouble determining which are your Top 3 or 5, let's talk at: www.sexyleanandstrong.com!

Step 3 – How to Strengthen, Repair and Prepare

Strengthen, repair and prepare guidelines – correcting your top three to five problems. Follow these guidelines for at least one week. See how much better you feel! When you have the strength and stamina, you can start down the mountain.

Water: one-half your weight in ounces per day (eg: I weigh 142 pounds, so I need at least 71 oz daily), taken throughout the day:

- One 8 oz. glass on rising
- One glass with ½ lemon juiced into it (adding cayenne or stevia are optional)
- One glass after breakfast
- The rest throughout the day, plus one glass about 2 hours before retiring (if heart problems run in the family, drink one glass of water one hour before you go to bed and keep some by the bed)

Sleep: 7 to 8 hours; prerequisites:

- Stop eating three hours before bed
- Get in some good exercise during the day
- Eat light for dinner
- Eat food with calcium and magnesium or take a supplement
- Use melatonin

Healthy Breakfast: consumed 12 hours after last meal/snack

- Lean proteins, protein shakes, eggs, plant-based proteins, approximately 250 to 450 calories, depending on your needs

Fiber: fruits, whole grains – 35 to 50 grams a day

- Pump-up nutrition with supplements and more veggies; Drop any sodas, candy, cookies, starches

Get Sufficient Protein: 10 to 15 grams at snack time and 20 to 40 grams at a meal; total recommended protein intake will depend on your weight, muscle mass and activity level -- See Appendix I – Dietary Programs

Limit Caffeine: to one serving, in the morning

Exercise: 30 minutes a day – brisk walking is fine

Stop eating three hours prior to bed

Add Probiotics: 4B minimum daily – best strains for longevity in your gut, per Dr. Wentz, are: Bifidobacterium BB-12 and Lactobacillus rhamnosus.

Limit Alcohol: Give the liver a break and only drink one or two glasses for this week or two. Alcohol is actually poison to the body and, if you are already struggling, you need to really reduce this for a period of time.

Differences Between Men and Women

These recommendations are applicable to both men and women – human cells are human cells! Where the differences come in is in the aging process – what hormones are depleting and what effect it is having on the body. Exercise strategies may vary slightly, but both sexes need cardio, strength-training, and stretching to stay lean and strong.

For the man over 50, there can be a lessening of the sex-drive due to lowered testosterone. For this, you will want to see your physician. I would not order just any testosterone-boosting agent or new pill from the radio or internet. There are just too few safeguards and too many risks due to lack of controls. Working out will help your body trigger more testosterone production, along with reducing the cortisol and helping to manage calories and cravings. Exercise and watching caloric intake late in the day will allow for restful sleep and keep the stress down.

Another area of concern for men, after the age of 50, is the health of the prostate gland. Taking the right supplements can support this area. I discuss these in the supplements recommendations in Step 4: "Discover Your Optimal Nutrition – Supplements and Why You Need Them".

For lagging energy, many of my male clients swear by Co-enzyme,Q10, which is the enzyme that provides the energy for all cells. This enzyme depletes over time and we cannot get it from food. It is critical for heart health and the health of the mitochondria, found in every cell.

Just like women, men have to manage their alcohol, sugar, caffeine and processed-food intake. They may be able to tolerate more alcohol due to heavier body-mass, but the liver is still having to work over-time and the belly will store the excess as fat.

My male clients have all wanted the same things as my female clients: more energy, less fat, more muscle, clean up the digestion, get rid of aches and pains and sleep better. They are given the same instructions as the gals – get rid of everything that is making your body mad: eat clean, exercise daily, drink your water, sleep enough to be fully-rested, give yourself some down-time!!! And, take some supplements to fill the gaps or help with extreme conditions.

Calorie Guidelines

Although I don't count calories, and rarely have my clients do so, it is still important to understand that you need to manage portion control and total calorie count over a day. Here are some guidelines from the National Institute for Aging, defined for adults over 50:

A woman over 50 who is:

- Not physically active needs about 1600 calories a day
- Somewhat physically active needs about 1800 calories a day
- Very active needs about 2000 calories a day

A man over 50 who is:

- Not physically active needs about 2000 calories a day
- Somewhat physically active needs about 2200-2400 calories a day
- Very active needs about 2400-2800 calories a day

Once we achieve our optimal weight, we need to manage our calories and exercise to maintain it. It is easy if you eat nutrient-dense food with lots of fiber and some healthy fats.

Chapter 3 –
Picking Up the Pieces

Living alone for the first time in almost my entire life, at 51, was gut-wrenching. I would try to find ways to calm myself and get to sleep. I tried to eat but the thought of food made me nauseous. I could not even smell it. I turned to the protein shake meal-replacements from my company and they not only stayed down but they took off the last few pounds.

Finally I was learning to take care of myself. I would get up and exercise, drink my shake, take my supplements, drink my water and look for someone to help. I was trying to keep my ranch going, learning to date for the first time in over thirty years, selling the family home, and running my nutrition products business. All at the same time, plus trying unsuccessfully to re-connect and build a relationship with my daughter.

After six months I was starting to feel I could handle it and then, at midnight on October 15, 2003, my ex called. My son Abe had died while at his birth-mother's home, at the age of 19 years, 10 months, of an accidental drug overdose. Everything just crashed down on me. I wanted the comfort of my ex but that was not an option.

My family and friends rallied around. I tried to keep the nutrition business going, but the first few weeks after Abe died, I was pretty non-functional. Luckily, by that time, I had a small team and they stepped-up and filled in for me.

Once our home sold I used the funds to move to another city. I needed to start over. My apartment had been two blocks from our home and it was too upsetting to drive past our block to get to my apartment. I needed to just be me, somewhere else. I needed to start over.

I took a consulting job back in high-tech. I made some good money and put it into a Florida real-estate investment. I sold the ranch and was dating a few guys. There was someone I had met early on that intrigued me, but we were maintaining a platonic relationship. Then, just before I moved out of the apartment, we got serious. Our relationship was pretty intense and we ended up in an on-again, off-again cycle for three years.

At one stage, during an off-cycle, I fell into a whirlwind romance and became engaged to someone else. Not only did I loan him money to pay off a debt, I helped him launch a home restoration/remodeling business by co-signing for a truck and a business credit card. Just as everything was percolating along, we broke up. He left the state, declaring bankruptcy, leaving me responsible for the debts. One month later, my Florida real-estate investment went bust, my partner backed-out and I had to pay-off the construction loan. I went from riches to rags in just months!

I was getting a lot of Life Lessons in a very short time! It was as though my early life was the charmed one and now I was paying for it with a ten year period of stress and struggle.

I had to stay strong, healthy and take care of myself. Emotionally, I was depleted and worn-out, but, I just focused on getting up every day, following my self-care process, and looking for someone to help. At the back of my mind, I struggled with having lost both my children – one to death and one who would have nothing to do with me.

My last Mother's Day with a child in my presence was May, 2002, when both Abe and Raquele were with me at the ranch. Since then, I am lucky if I get a phone call on Mother's Day. I used to dread the day, but lately I have been able to handle it without getting depressed, by telling myself that I did the best I could and I have nothing to blame myself for.

There are several "anniversary" days that create stress and tension in my body. Mother's Day, October 15th -- the day my son died, Valentine's day (our kids moved in on Valentine's Day, my divorce papers arrived on Valentine's Day, twelve years later, and I put down my beloved companion, Boomer, on February 13, 2014). I find my body starts getting tense and I start not sleeping and feeling sick. I have to focus on getting all the right foods, not turning to the old comfort foods – candy, chips, bread, ice cream -- and getting daily exercise – the kind that makes you sweat and breathe hard. I have to do the yoga and deep breathing and self-care. I have to stay positive and focus on the good in my life. I still have some weepy times during those anniversaries, but I am getting better.

When I have clients with these types of "anniversaries", we design a plan to keep them sane and healthy. Keeping busy is key, and staying on the right foods and limiting the alcohol. You also need to make sure you have someone to talk to, who will let you express your sadness and just love you through it!

During these anniversaries, you need the support of good friends. These are the kind with whom you can weep and carry on, or go out and get into some fun activity, just to keep your mind off the memory and distract yourself from the emotions flooding through your body.

Without my friends, I could not have weathered all I did and come out strong at the end.

Chapter 4 –
Building A New Life

By 2006, the divorce was final. I was living alone and back seeing my on-again, off-again beau. He was persistent and loving and we decided to take a stab at living together. I moved in, and we went through a major adjustment cycle for several months, with some rather intense arguments. We were such different people, with totally different backgrounds. While I was a college graduate, a white-collar worker, from upper-management, he was in the construction industry and had dropped out of college to marry and take care of his son. He had been in the same city his entire life – fifty-five years. He had friends he had known all his life. I had been a nomad. As a child, I attended thirteen elementary schools and, as an adult, had moved every six to seven years. He was most comfortable with routine -- things, people and places he knew. I wanted constant change and excitement and was used to being in a new place and learning to adapt.

He had lived alone, in the same home, for over thirty-four years, raising his son as a single-parent, and dating many women. I had been with one man since I was nineteen and was married to him for almost thirty years. We both had certain expectations, which turned out to be completely opposite. The home was quite small and, with my business booming, we were feeling confined. He was commuting to a job over sixty miles away and working long hours, including weekends. We were ships passing in the night. Yet, despite it all, I knew I loved him and he kept telling me he would never leave me. Finally, we took the plunge and married in a simple ceremony on the beach in Kauai, in May of 2007.

By 2009 we were in a new home together, a gorgeous custom, five-bedroom sprawling and spacious home with a pool, near his job. We were living in a brand-new town, where I had no connections. I had to make a new life. I joined the local Chamber of Commerce, started networking and made new friends. I kept my team going by traveling back to the old stomping-grounds, but it took at least four hours a day, round-trip. Gradually my team grew their own leadership and I could focus on building locally.

The marriage was challenging and adjusting to each other's needs took us to marriage counselors and through several books on relationships and relating. I meet and work with many divorcees, who are struggling with the dating scene and new relationships. It has been helpful to have my own struggles to share with them. Again, it is as though I am supposed to learn everything about life in the years I have left so I can bring it to bear when needed.

As part of the journey to the new life, I have gone through a lot of education and training, along with some personal development course-work. Some of the work was done in weekend seminars, others in years-long courses. All have allowed me to bring thousands of hours of study and work together to help my clients and now, hopefully, you.

First, I went through the Klemmer and Associates program for personal development, graduating the Samurai Camp and becoming a Sam Camp group facilitator. Here we learned what we are driven by, how we come across to others, and how to set lofty goals and achieve them. We learned how to Mastermind and work as a team to bring our group energy to bear on a problem. Mostly, we learned to tune in to ourselves and be true to our real natures. I had to stop lying to myself or hiding the fact that I was a "tough cookie" and learn to soften. My name at Klemmer was "brass-knuckles". The hardest word I had to take on was "gentle". In my life, being gentle meant being walked-on or beaten-up. I would start swinging the brass-knuckles before that could happen. It cost me big in my first marriage, and with my children. It is something I have to work at every day now. I focus on trying to sense what is going on with the other person and not jump to a fight before I get the full story.

Ultimately I have had to acknowledge and admit to myself that I was a big factor in why my first marriage broke-up, and I alienated my daughter. I have had to do a lot of soul-searching to realize I was letting my emotions get away from me. I never realized how painful I was making it for my children and husband.

The second most important education I went through was the training at several institutions and certification programs in fitness and nutrition. First was the American Fitness Professionals Association, where I certified as a Nutrition and Wellness Consultant. Next was a holistic hospital and health resort, Sanoviv Medical Institute, where I certified as a Nutrition and Wellness Advisor, specializing in digestion, detox and diabetes. Finally, my training with the Institute for Integrative Nutrition as a Certified Integrative Health Coach, studying nutrition and over one hundred dietary theories, so that I have the ability to determine what is going on and what needs to change to help you get off the mountain.

I encourage everyone going through life-changes, loss and struggles to add something new to your life – music lessons, crafts, studies, traveling, new groups. Build a new life and make it yours! Find new things and people to excite and motivate you. Do not wallow in the self-pity and eat yourself into a coma, trying to soothe what is troubling you. Seek out counselors and coaches, read books, journal on your thoughts. The emotions must be acknowledged and addressed for you to achieve your happiness. I had to work through complete loss and desolation, to be able to feel I was still worthy of love, that I had something to offer and that my life was not over because I had lost my best friend and lover of over thirty years. I was not worthless because I could not save my son, and my daughter would not talk to me. I had to know there was something I could do to give back.

You need to do the same. You need to stay vital, sexy, lean and strong for yourself! It does not matter how old you are, you can always learn something new that can take you away from your troubles. Volunteer, visit the elderly and infirm, teach kids to read. Do something so you know you are still of value and have something to give back. Help those who are worse off than you. Live with gratitude for your life, body and mind.

Chapter 5 –
Chart Your Path Off the Mountain

Who are you, what do you want to be, do, and have, and what will it take to make this happen?

Getting off the mountain successfully requires really understanding who you are, what you want to be, do, and have, and what it will take to make this happen. There are many factors you have to address. Remember, just calorie-counting is not going to do it. To discover your path will mean some real digging. It is buried deep inside you and we have to draw it out. You are going to go on a self-discovery journey, which will ultimately tell you how to get off the mountain. We are going to do this together, piece by piece, until there is a plan that will work for you.

Dealing with all the new stuff – home, marriage, studying and new career, brought a lot of questions and self-analysis. It was very helpful to me to realize that who I am today-- mentally, physically and emotionally— was, to some extent, determined before I was even born. When we come into the world, we are a product of our parents, grandparents and all their DNA. The term here is "bio-individuality" – we are all unique individuals – we have human DNA, but we also have our own specific genes, built from our mother and our father and their specific genes, passed down from generations.

Our emotions and ability to handle stress or extreme feelings, is driven by how we were brought up, what we learned at home and at school and church. Watching others we admired and loved melt-down, like my mom, or walk-out and never contact you, like my dad, shaped who I am today. Who I am today drives how I act and thus, my emotional state, which also drives my chemistry and how I process my food.

The Chemistry of the Mad Body

So many times our emotions drive our behaviors, especially eating. When we are happy, sad, depressed, anxious, angry, tense, stressed, frustrated, confused -- a lot of us eat. And we don't always eat something healthy – we eat something we know is not good for us but that fits that hunger to feel better, usually something that soothed us as a child – ice cream, cookies, chips, peanut butter on crackers, candy. Mindfulness goes out the window and we simply fill the hole in our heart. Until we make ourselves sick and then get mad at ourselves, and then eat again to calm that down, creating the vicious cycle that puts us on Mad-Body Mountain.

Emotions and understanding what they do to us is key. As Candice Pert, PhD, says in "Molecules of Emotion", "The chemicals that are running our body and our brain are the same chemicals that are involved in emotion. And it says to me that....we'd better pay more attention to emotions with respect to health."

The Chemistry
of the *Mad-Body*

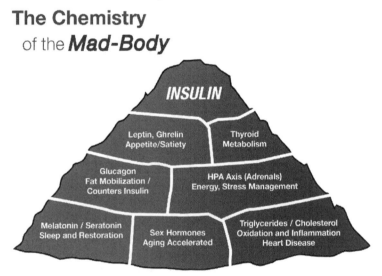

Our chemistry is so important and in our power to manage, but most of just ignore it and take it for granted. Chemists and biologists will tell you our bodies are all about our chemistry. What you eat is what you are! What you think is how you eat! What you eat and create in terms of chemistry is how you feel. It is all connected and part of the Factors of the Mad-Body. If your chemistry is out-of-balance due to any of the factors, then the chemistry of the hormones and enzymes is sure to be off. Once you know you are out-of-balance, you then choose to Strengthen, Repair and Prepare or jump into your descent plan. It is all about what you are experiencing, right now!

Sometimes people are stuck in their childhood eating patterns, sometimes they are trying to eat healthy and not succeeding. Sometimes certain foods cause upset – emotionally and physically. There are a lot of factors that affect what we can and cannot eat comfortably. It can be chemistry – missing hormones, enzymes, probiotics, or intolerances and sensitivities all the way to allergies. It can be a result of operations and loss of organs or glands, or an ongoing illness. We have to eliminate the foods that create real discomfort and determine what we can eat that will actually nourish us at an optimal level, not just satisfy a craving or habit developed in childhood.

Often we go along with the bad eating choices of our significant other or family members because it is easier, or because we are actually addicted to the problem foods. In particular, you can be addicted to certain foods, but not all of them. There are two extremely addictive foods – sugar and flour. Sugar and flour both act in the body the same way – fast metabolization, leaving you wanting more of the same thing. For some, sugar and flour are as addictive as alcohol and cocaine. They hit the same pleasure-centers in the brain and we crave more after they run-out. You know yourself. Be honest and walk away from them if they present a problem.

There are several key factors that play a role in our food choices and reactions to food today: blood type, race, origin, health of our parents at the time of conception, and then what our mother ate and drank, felt and did while we were in-utero, and whether we were born vaginally or by caesarean. Another factor is whether we were breast or bottle-fed. All of these factors contribute to the basic human body we start with. Then, you add all the years and all the food, stress, exercise, injuries, illness, love, or lack of, that turn us into who we are.

You may be surprised to find out that your family history and heritage is only twenty per-cent of what causes your health. The rest is what you have done to that perfect body since you were born. What you have thought, been taught and told, what you ate, breathed, drank, smoked, ingested, how you were treated, what physical activity you had and how much sleep you got. It all factors in.

Once you have done the work to determine what stage you are, and what brought you there, then it is up to you (and maybe a health coach or other support person), to figure out the ideal plan to bring you down the mountain.

Factor in who you were, who you are today and who you want to be. Set realistic goals, create a tracking process, reward yourself when you do well and re-commit when you go backwards.

You are not going to get off this mountain except one step at a time! No leaping to the bottom. There will be times when you can run for a bit, safely, and then you will have to slow down again to navigate a treacherous path. Now, you are up to Step 4 in the Planning process.

Step 4 – Discover Your Optimal Nutrition Strategy

What should you eat? How is your digestion? Do you need to detox? Cleanse? Fast? What supplements do you need?

How do you find out which foods are upsetting you when you have been eating pretty much the same things for years? You become your own "mad-scientist". Think of yourself as an experiment. One way is to try an Elimination Diet to find the foods you should not eat and all the good foods you can eat.

Elimination Diet Instructions

Go twenty-three days without:

- Gluten, dairy, eggs, corn, soy, fast food, any foods you are already allergic to, or alcohol.

Note: Gluten is found in wheat, rye, and barley.

What can you eat?

- 30% "clean" protein, i.e. organic, hormone-free, grass-fed, happy, lean beef, chicken, and wild fish and shellfish (unless you are allergic)
- 70% vegetables, legumes (think beans and lentils), nuts, seeds, seaweeds, and gluten-free grains like quinoa

DO. . .

- DO eat fish. (But watch out for high mercury-content fish such as tuna and swordfish.)
- DO eat lots of fiber, fresh whole foods, and unprocessed meals you make yourself.
- DO eat lots of healthy fats found in olive oil, ghee, coconut oil, sunflower oil, flax oil, walnut oil, and avocados.

DO NOT. . .

- Do NOT carbo load on gluten-free breads, cereals and crackers.

Continue all supplements and drink lemon water on rising. Stick with your exercise schedule and make sure you get enough sleep – 7 to 8 hours per night.

Next, reintroduce the eliminated foods, one at a time. This is how:

On day twenty-four, pick one thing you eliminated—like gluten, OR dairy, OR eggs—but not more than one, and eat it, at each meal – that day.

See how you feel over the next 48 hours. If you have no reaction after two days, eat that same food again, and for a second time, notice how you feel. From there, it's up to you whether or not to re-incorporate that food into your diet on a regular basis.

Once you've made a call on the first food you reintroduce, pick another one and follow the same steps. Throughout the diet and the reintroduction process, notice how you feel. Maybe you'll see changes you weren't expecting. Maybe your sleep quality or your energy level is better. Maybe the redness in your skin is gone, or your belly is flatter.

Finding out what life without a particular food will be like means you could be saving yourself a lifetime of inflammation, annoying symptoms, and in some cases, even life-threatening diseases.

Evaluate: What did you find out? What foods give you the most energy? What foods disturb you in some way? And now, what should you eat? The list of foods that your body will love is super-important as that is the basis of your new lifestyle and how you are going to get down the mountain.

Blood-Type Discussion

After the Elimination Diet phase, sometimes there is still an issue and the weight will not come off. Here is where I add in the advice from Eat Right for Your Type, by Dr. Peter D'Adamo. His reasoning is that certain foods carry specific proteins and these can be a mismatch for our blood proteins, which can cause weight-gain even if the calorie count is right. I found that, as a Blood Type B -- I do better with some free-range, organic animal protein, fish, lots of vegetables, some nuts, very little grains, sugar or dairy. Quite Paleo, as it turns out. My blood-type needs lots of protein to stay lean and have stamina. For me, living mostly Paleo, it is quite easy to stay lean, without really focusing on it. (See the list of some of the most popular diet-styles and their definitions in the Appendices.)

Though nothing is 100% applicable to everyone, especially in light of our susceptibility to cravings and our willpower, still it is helpful to understand which blood type we are and take a look at the guidelines. After doing an elimination diet, adding back in foods that are deemed "wrong" for our blood type can create issues. Living with any one system or guideline for 90 days will tell you a lot.

Getting the Right Food to Your Plate

Now that you have determined what foods are best for you and what foods you want to eat the most of, you have to make it appear on a plate! I don't always have time to cook, but I can still eat healthfully and quickly using my process of Acquire, Assemble, Consume. I buy packages of greens, or prepared full-meal salads, plus lean proteins or fish, fresh organic veggies and fruit, organic eggs, and then do the least amount of prep possible. I love green smoothies, steamed veggies and veggie stir-frys and soups! Things I can put together quickly and that are super-healthy. Then, if the rest of the family is not into that food, or eating foods that are a problem for me, I have something good for me.

I stay away from GMO foods and processed anything, 90% of the time. My body is the happiest, leanest and strongest it has been in years!

Some of my clients are body-builders and fitness models. They will get within twelve weeks of a competition and pound down three chicken breasts a day, some fish, plus some brown rice or oatmeal, and vegetables – asparagus, broccoli, green beans. They consume no sugar, including fruit, and, right before competition, cut their water consumption back. We don't have to be so severe, but, if we model this type of eating, most of us can lean down very quickly.

If you love to cook, have the time, and are feeding a family, there are many great cookbooks out there. I love Low-Glycemic Meals in Minutes because there is a good variety and they have lots of great family-style dishes. Just let yourself be guided by what you are trying to accomplish. If you need to feed more than one or two, it takes a bit more planning. I like the concept of prepping the meats and vegetables on Sunday, so you can make meals all week. Get the kids and spouse involved so it becomes a fun activity and you don't feel like the little house-maid. The key is to plan the week's meals, plus snacks, and then stick with the plan! It is the unplanned "treats" and extra food that does us in and keeps us up on the mountain.

Once your food-style is nailed down, you are going to want to make sure you are getting all the nutrition you need to and are staying non-toxic. Here is where we move to the Digestion, Elimination and Detoxing discussion.

Digestion, Elimination and Detoxing

Many of the enzymes and hormones that support our body's nutrition absorption and cleansing processes are reduced with the passage of time. To think we can eat after 50 the way we did at age 20 or 30 is wrong and the body will soon get "upset" and "angry" when we try to do so. Many choose to subdue the body's natural responses to too much oil, fat, and artificial sweeteners and other additives, then take over-the-counter solutions for acid reflux and indigestion, because it is easier. Easier than listening to our mad body, acknowledging we are making the wrong choices, and taking steps to correct them.

There are many good ways to clean up the digestive system. Laying off the junk foods, adding in probiotics and digestive enzymes, chewing our food enough (35 times per bite, till you have mush, not lumps), drinking less alcohol, eating less animal protein, eating smaller portions, drinking more water. If you have an upset tummy, acid reflux, Irritable Bowel Syndrome, constipation, gas and bloating, you need to fix your digestion and strengthen the liver and gut, not take something to shut your body up or close down natural processes!

Living for years on antacids or acid-blockers can weaken your immune system and mask the real cause of the issue. Try some of the natural solutions along with the medication. Never quit any medication cold-turkey without checking with your health-care practitioner! Although food is medicine and medicine is food, we have to take into consideration there can be interactions between the medicines and certain foods and supplements. But, if you want to add some natural help, here are some tips:

You can eat fermented vegetables, greek yogurt, drink probiotic-rich beverages, take probiotic, liver and digestive enzyme supplements, drink bone broth, make healthy meals and lay-off the processed and unhealthy foods. Do this for about three weeks and see what your body tells you. Just three days of doing this and the liver will already have begun restoring itself! Two weeks and you will feel and look like a younger you! A side benefit will be clearer skin and losing weight!

Cleanses and Fasts – Should you do one and which to do when?

Fatty foods, rich meats, quantities of dairy, too many flour-based foods, alcohol, toxins, stress, medicines, sugar and lack of exercise all serve to upset the older body. Cleansing or fasting can help get it back on-track. If you have never done a cleanse or fast, don't just jump into one. I feel you must go through the Strengthen, Repair and Prepare phase to be able to get through one successfully.

After doing SRP at least one week, possibly as much as one month, your body and mind are prepared and you can think about doing a cleanse or jump-start diet to take some weight off fast. This helps get you motivated for the climb down. Many lose weight just making the changes during the SRP phase!

The majority benefit from cleanses and fasts, when done right and for the right reasons. Diets don't work, because they are too rigid and call for willpower, which cannot be maintained permanently. Cleanses are temporary and can help the body kick sugar and carbohydrate addictions, setting you up for better body chemistry and control over your cravings. They can also give you a jump-start on losing weight, which boosts morale and gets you committed to continue. Until you get control, it can be really hard to implement all the changes you need to.

I put my clients on a cleanse or mini-fast when I see that their system is so overloaded from too many poor meals, stress or bad eating habits that it just needs an overhaul. Unless we are doing a major cleanse, it won't last more than five to seven days, and it needs to be structured around enough protein, carbs, fats and fiber to keep them full and satisfied. They also need to get enough nutrients to curb cravings.

The studies are clear that liquid meal-replacement shakes are a great way to lose weight, and fast! But, we don't want to live on them. If you are getting less than 1000 calories a day, then it might back-fire and you could end up with the starvation response. Over time you will gain all the weight back because you won't have a way to eat real food without overdoing it. You have to incorporate healthy choices after you complete a cleanse.

Choosing a cleanse program can be a daunting task! There are many good cleanses out there. Different experts and coaches will have their own recommendations. I have my preferred cleanse products and I have great success with my clients. When selecting meal-replacement shakes, look for products that have good science behind them. Low sugar (natural, not artificial) , high-fiber, with enough protein and calories to keep you satisfied (around 240 to 300 calories per serving and 80 to100 grams of protein a day, depending on weight and activity level). I also recommend gluten-free formulas and of course, organic and non-GMO.

Cleanses

Standard, short-term Cleanse Options: Juicing, Fruit, Protein and high-fiber, Vegan

Simple Cleanse: Cutting out all starch and processed foods

Works for Stage 1 – Upset and most of Stage 2 – Angry

- Limit sugar to natural sugars and no more than 40 grams per day. No fake sugars!
- Increase good fats -- olive, avocado, hemp, flax, coconut oil to two servings a day, about 2 tsp or half of an avocado
- Drink enough water (half your weight in ounces a day)
- Get enough sleep (7 to 8 hours a night, every night, for one week minimum)
- Eat right for your body (blood-type, heritage, culture, environ-ment, gut)
- Add Fiber (35 to 50 grams a day) and Probiotics (4B a day)
- Get Enough Protein – lean, organic, 80 to 100 grams a day
- Add Probiotics – 4B a day, minimum

Major Cleanses

These are used to get the Stage 2 and 3 body back on-track. They have to be chosen carefully and then managed to determine if there are any adverse effects. They can be very effective, but I would advise getting a professional involved if you have never experienced one. Cleanses do promote eliminating, and can have detox effects – headaches, joint pain, nausea, light-headedness. I recommend working with someone who has used it before and understands what you are going through, so they can tweak the program to resolve any issues.

Liver, full detox – 7 to 60 days

Detox and Heal Your Liver – Getting your liver healthy equals easier fat-loss. Which detox you use is the key – a great one is The Liver Cleanse Diet by Dr. Sandra Cabot. You need to dedicate eight weeks for the full cycle. The first phase is two weeks where you ease your body into the limitations. Then, four weeks on a restricted list of permitted foods, and then two weeks to finish up. This is what I used with Marnie, and it worked! You can actually live on the foods used in the middle phase, in fact, I do! They meet all my needs and I feel great and don't gain weight.

Here is a quick summary of what to expect:

- Better sleep
- Clearer skin
- More and easier elimination
- Energy to burn!
- Reduced belly-fat
- Less cravings
- Reduced food allergies
- Weight-loss

You can also help your liver with some supplements: milk-thistle, alpha-lipoic acid, turmeric.

Colon Cleanses – Two to Three Days

You can eat to cleanse the colon, drink to cleanse the colon, use enemas and get hydro-colonics (wash it out with water). I recommend colon cleansing when the body is dealing with built-up gunk from years of being bad – processed foods, no probiotics, lots of animal protein, little exercise. It can be great to let your body get truly empty and cleaned-out. (Prepping for a colonoscopy does this, but, it is N-A-S-T-Y!) With a colon cleanse diet, you can eat or drink things that are not nauseating. Cleansing the colon allows you to get rid of major toxic-buildup and restores good gut-bacteria for better nutrition absorption.

Colon cleansing involves fiber, lots of greens, lots of good fats, probiotics, and flushing with water. Plan the timing carefully! Since you are cleansing the colon, you need to be where you can get to a restroom quickly. You might plan to stay home for the two or three days. After the cleanse make sure you re-inoculate your colon with good probiotics to speed-up the recovery.

Fasting

There are fasts that last from 24 hours all the way to 30 days. When fasting, you limit your calories to very low, or you take in no food at all. A "pure" fast (as used at the Bragg Institute) is to drink only distilled water, with an optional splash of lemon juice, eight to ten glasses a day. Some add cranberry juice drops to some bubbly-water, others add maple syrup or cayenne.

Other "fasts" will be based on just bone or vegetable broth, or drinking the lemon juice/water all day with just a light vegetable meal in the afternoon. The point is to give the body a break from all the processing and eliminating and really clean it out. Fasting has shown some amazing benefits. The lightness of being that results is amazing! The organs are so grateful for the break from processing food and the blood is revitalized. Make sure to pick a very light-activity day when you can really benefit from the cleansing process. Rest afterwards, take a nice relaxing bath and go to bed early!

I practice and recommend "intermittent fasting"– taking in no food for the twelve hours between dinner and breakfast. This is highly beneficial for the liver and kidneys and will help to get a flat belly in no time! If you eat really late at night, just don't load up again in the morning until a full 12 hours have passed since the dinner.

Another strategy is to do one 24-hour fast weekly. Again, the goal is to rest the organs and give the body time to repair without having to constantly process, digest and assimilate food. It is all about you and what you want to accomplish. Check with your health-care professional before trying a fast, especially a long one (more than three days, in fact).

"Pure" Fasting, what it is and how to do it (per the Bragg Institute):

Consume absolutely no food, drinking only eight to ten glasses of distilled water each day of the fast. The length of time varies; it is up to you and your tolerance and goals. The recommendation is to start with one or two days, then work your way up to more, as your body becomes accustomed. How long you go depends on what you want to accomplish, how toxic you are and how long it takes to clean your body up.

Benefits: clear-head, clear-body, clear-skin, weight loss

Pros: cleans out the organs, releases salt, inorganic minerals, heavy metals, fat.

Cons: Hunger, fatigue, detox symptoms – headaches, muscle and joint aches, stomach aches, the runs

Process: Eat clean and light (1200 calories a day -- mostly vegan) for three to four days prior, then do distilled water only for 24 to 36 hours. Eat super-clean for two days after; starting with vegetable broth.

Keep track of how you feel during all the phases – prep, during and after – this will tell you a lot about what your body wants. Again, involve your physician if you are on medication, or are being seen for any health issues.

Supplements and Why You Need Them

As I tell my clients, "You can't get it all from food." (Unless you consume four different green/red/brown/blue smoothies a day with nine servings of different vegetables and the right amount and type of protein!) RDAs (U.S. Government Recommended Daily Amounts) of nutrients will not come close to what we need today to combat all the toxins we are dealing with. They cannot stop degenerative diseases such as cancer, heart disease, arthritis, diabetes. They can't even prevent colds and flus! All they will do is keep us from getting nutrient-deficient diseases such as scurvy and rickets. They are a minimal amount of nutrition, a poverty-level way of nourishing our bodies. But, if we need more, then how are we going to get it?

Once upon a time real food had enough nutrients that our parents and grandparents could be properly nourished with a healthy diet. Now, even if we could eat enough, the food is not powerful enough (depletion by corporate-farming, mono-crop, no rotation, nutrient-depleted soil, not to mention pesticides, herbicides and GMO foods) – supplementing closes the gaps and gives us the nutrition we need to stay energized and lean.

There are a lot of key nutrients we need, every day. For example, we should get 400 IU of Vitamin E a day (the RDA is 40 IU.) To get this from a food source would mean eating three pounds of almonds, for a total of 8,900 calories, or, thirty-three pounds of spinach! As I cannot possibly eat that much food a day, I find it much easier to add the vitamins and supplement program to close the gaps. It is much easier and cheaper than spending large sums of money on bushels of fresh produce, along with all the juicing, chewing and digesting to meet all the body's daily needs for optimal nutrition.

Maintaining Healthy Hormonal Levels

Hormones are the chemical messengers that control our emotions, chemistry and cravings, weight and just about everything in the body. Two main hormones are insulin and adrenaline. If your hormones are out-of-whack, kiss the new eating plan good-bye! There are many good ways to help a body with changing hormones from aging, surgeries or medication. In addition to getting rid of processed and GMO foods, and adding green smoothies and plant protein, enough water, and sleep, my clients use the products offered by my nutrition company as they work extremely well. The key is to make sure you are addressing the right symptoms with the right solution. Most important is to get checked-out by a doctor who specializes in hormonal imbalances. Sometimes it is the right thing to get on some hormonal supplements, which need to come from a medical source. Often-times, the reports come back border-line and it is left up to you to find a natural, safe way to support your body's changing needs.

Each age has its own challenges in terms of changing and declining hormones. In our 40s, most women move into menopause, when the progesterone, testosterone and estrogen begin to decrease. With less progesterone comes aches and pains in the joints, chronic fatigue, depression, sleep disturbances, weight gain and anxiety.

By age 50, the thyroid begins to strain and DHEA levels begin to decrease. Men may begin to experience Andropause (the male version of menopause). Both men and women go through a decline in hormones, namely testosterone. Women not through with menopause will continue with estrogen and progesterone fluctuations. When the thyroid function starts to decline, you may lose your hair, experience weight gain, become constipated, become hypertensive (increased blood pressure), feel sluggish and demotivated. You can get some support naturally with Tyrosine, Iodine and Kelp.

In the 60s, the body's ability to cope with sugar declines and the insulin resistance or diabetes becomes more prevalent. Typical middle-age spread is due to the fact that the hormones no longer protect the body from the bad effects of the spikes and dips in the sugar levels.

The good news is this is all reversible with the right nutrition and supplements!

Enzymes and What They Do

Enzymes are involved in every process of the body. Enzymes digest all of our food and make it small enough to pass through the tiniest pores of the intestines into the blood. Enzymes in the blood take the prepared, digested food and build it into muscles, nerves, blood, organs and glands. The number of enzymes in the body is overwhelming and each one has a specific function. How do you get enzymes? Some are found in foods. Some we are born with, cannot make more of and lose with age. The more enzyme-deficient we are, the faster we age.

If you are lacking in certain enzymes, you may not be able to digest certain foods. If you are experiencing gas or bloating or indigestion, you need to think about adding more vegetables and fruit, particularly raw vegetables. Enzymes are very fragile and are destroyed at high temperatures.

There are four categories of food enzymes. They are:

1. Lipase – which serves to break down fat
2. Protease – works to break down protein
3. Cellulase – assists in breaking down cellulose
4. Amylase – which breaks down starch

But the need for enzymes goes beyond digestive processes. There are three major classes of enzymes: metabolic enzymes (enzymes which work in blood, tissues, and organs), food enzymes from raw food, and digestive enzymes. Our organs are run by metabolic enzymes. These enzymes take food substances and build them into healthy tissue and have numerous other duties. We need to remember that we inherited an enzyme reserve at birth and this quantity can be decreased as we age by eating an enzyme-deficient diet. One way this reserve is reduced is by eating most of our food cooked. Then, our digestive systems have to produce all of the enzymes, which causes an enlargement of the digestive organs. The body will draw on its reserve from all organs and tissues, causing a metabolic deficit. The best way to fix this is eat more raw vegetables and, if necessary, take digestive enzyme supplements.

Supplements We All Need to Counteract Aging and Poor Food Choices

Women:

- Multi-vitamin/chelated mineral supplements
- Calcium
- Fish-oil capsules
- Menstrual symptom support
- Probiotics
- Digestive Enzymes

Men:

- Multi-vitamins/chelated minerals
- Fish-oil capsules
- Prostate support
- Probiotics
- Digestive Enzymes

The main support will come from balancing all the bodily functions with the advanced cellular nutrition in the multi-vitamins, minerals, probiotics, fish fatty-acid Omega-3s and the melatonin sleep-aid. These go a long way to helping the client with hormonal fluctuations due to aging or chronic illness to regain vigor and a happy attitude.

Key Supplements

Sex Hormones: estrogen, progesterone, testosterone – bio-identical forms, through a doctor; or, herbal supplements to help lessen the effects of the changes

Age-Depleted Hormones: HGH, DHEA, serotonin, TSH

Age-Depleted Enzymes: Co-enzyme Q10

Digestive Enzymes: amylase, protease, bromelian, papain

Antoxidants: bioflavonoids, polyphenols

Vitamins: A – as beta-carotene, B-2, B-6, B-12, riboflavin, niacin, thiamin, C, D, E – pure, not synthetic, K

Minerals: calcium, phosphorus, silicon, boron, vanadium, magnesium, manganese, copper, selenium, zinc,

Joint Support: glucosamine, turmeric

Vision Support: Omega-3, Vitamin A as beta-carotene, lycopene, zeaxanthin, bilberry

Immune System: Vitamin C, Vitamin D-3, grapeseed extract, turmeric, enzymes

Probiotics: multiple strains, 4B minimum daily, get the kind that survive the stomach acid

Prebiotics: fiber that feeds the probiotics (whole grains, vegetables, psyllium, whole fruit)

Fish-fatty acids: Omega-3s--for brain, muscle, heart

Multi-vitamin/mineral system: bio-available, pharmaceutical-grade, compounded products that guarantee the dosage and combination for synergy and effectiveness

Menopause support: Soy isoflavones, chasteberry, licorice, dong quai, black cohosh, wild yam, evening primrose

Prostate support: saw palmetto, lycopene, soy isoflavones

Choosing a Supplement Company/Product

- Find out what Manufacturing standards they use – you want USP (pharmaceutical-grade) not USDA (food-grade)
- Manufacturing facility location and operation
- Source and type of ingredients –- organic, country-of-origin
- What guarantees are they providing – purity, potency, disinte-

gration, bioavailability, absorption rate

- What 3rd party certifications do they have – such as: Consumer-Labs, FDA-registered facility, NSF for Sport, Physicians Desk Reference on Medicine
- Ranking in the Comparative Guide to Nutritional Supplements—see References
- Customer Service and customer satisfaction rankings

If you are going to get your body in top-shape to get down the mountain, you have to take the right supplements that are formulated to do the job, that will really make a difference. My clients and I have great results with the suppliers I have listed in the Resources. There are many good companies out there. Just make sure you invest in your health with a good line, not a cheap imitation off a grocery-store or drug-store shelf, with little to no guarantees or quality-control!

Step 5 – Design Your Best Exercise Program

Remember – you can't exercise your way out of poor nutrition! All the exercise in the world does not matter if you are eating junk. You may have a firm body, but no real stamina, immunity or healthy gut.

You will need to determine how much exercise and what type will do the most for you, and what you can successfully do. Body type, bone structure, weight, blood-type, your physical condition and any injuries can be factors in this.

Lifestyle Factors to Consider

Too many people join a gym and then, never go, or, they go, take a class, hire a trainer and then get hurt and quit going. Pick something you can stick with and make it a daily practice. Have a variety of things you like so you do not get bored and your muscles do not get accustomed to the same thing. When your body is habituated to a particular exercise, the muscles don't work as hard so you don't burn calories as efficiently.

What is the right exercise program for you? Ask yourself: What fits your lifestyle? Sports, gym, at-home practice? Indoors, outdoors?

Alone, in a group? How much weight do you want to lose and what will help keep you toned and retain muscles? What to consider:

- How can you make it happen every day?
- How can you keep it interesting?

The Goal:

Exercise at least 30 minutes a day, every day—cardio and strengthen/tone – you can break this up into two fifteen-minute segments if you have a crazy schedule. But you have to get moving! Sitting is killing us; movement will save us!

Break a sweat, breathe hard and feel the burn, but don't get hurt!

See the Appendix for which exercises burn how many calories and have some fun! Even housework (and sex) count, so give yourself credit for stuff besides the normal pumping-iron or spin class.

Home-based or Gyms

Home-based programs – self-paced using DVDs, YouTube, television shows – these all work. You may need equipment and to set aside some space. My favorite at-home exercises include: rebounder, yoga, pilates, yoga-lates, kick-boxing, dancing, my Total Gym – just about anything and everything. Find things you love and change them up to keep your body engaged and responding.

Gyms – If you are using a gym, make sure you get checked-out on the equipment and work with a trainer a few times to get a good routine established. You can make-up your own routine, but I love the group classes for the ability to just focus on the effort and stop thinking about what I should be doing next. It is easier to get some direction and fun to be part of a group. Most of my clients in Stage 1 and 2 are fine with the gym. Clients in Stage 3 will often wait a few months to build up endurance, strength and confidence before going to a gym. Some trainers will come to your home. Wherever you are in the process, you must fit in the exercise!

Folks with Challenges

I have worked with folks in their late 60s all the way to 80 and obtained improvement. Sometimes they can only exercise while sitting in a chair, but you can get a lot of good muscle-action, even seated in a chair. The point is to move, no matter what your condition. You can even get blood-flowing and toxins moving out if you are bed-ridden. You can tighten parts of the body, breathing in and out, tensing and releasing the muscle. Work your way up from the feet to the head, tensing and releasing. Open and close hands and wiggle fingers and toes. Just move!

Building the Best Exercise Program for You

Different body types respond best to specific exercise programs. There are three main body types:

Pear: Pears, like me, gain and carry excess weight from the waist down, especially the belly, hips and thighs. Our waists can be quite small compared to the belly and hips. When out-of-shape, we have a small bust/chest, with an obvious waist, big belly and huge hips, thighs and butt. We respond best to extended sessions of sweat-producing cardio to start burning fat, plus good overall toning, with focus on building up the upper body. This helps us to lose belly-fat quickly. The HIT program works well for pears. (High-Intensity Interval Training -- 1 minute of exercise, 1 minute of rest, with six to seven exercises and 2 reps of the circuit)

Apple: Apples are round, from the chest/bust to waist and belly, the measurements all match within a few inches. The first two weeks of the program they will not see a lot of change, unless they are using a cleanse or fast. Most apple women are large-busted, with almost no perceptible waist and a belly that matches the waist. The hips and butt are small by comparison and they look quite top-heavy. The best exercises for Apples are overall body-conditioning with 20 minutes of cardio, working up to 45 minutes or more cardio and about 20 to 30 minutes of strength-training, every day. Abs will respond last, and to lose belly-fat takes concentrated effort along with literally no sugar and starch.

Curvy: The curvy figure is equally bodacious in bust and hips. The waist is much smaller in proportion, but, when this figure type is overweight, the belly and thighs will be quite large as well. Curvy types need a lot of exercise to trim down. They will want to do a minimum of 30 to 45 minutes of cardio, daily, plus 15 to 20 minutes of strength-training two to three times a week.

Here are some plans
that will work for all types:

Day 1 to Day 60 plan: *30-minutes a Day to Sexy, Lean and Strong*

- Flexibility – full-body stretches for 5 to 10 minutes a day
- Strength – do some weight-bearing exercises for about 10 to 12 minutes a day (push-ups, crunches, planks, machines)
- Endurance – running, fast walking, dancing, jumping rope, quick cycling for 12 minutes
- HIT – High Intensity Interval Training – great for breaking a sweat and getting a full workout in a short time (1 minute of exercise, 1 minute of rest, with six to seven exercises and 2 reps of the circuit) – can sub-in for the Endurance and Strength

Day 61 to Day 120 plan: *45-minutes a day to Even Sexier, Leaner and Stronger*

- Cardio/Stamina – 20 minutes of some movement – run, dance, walk, bike, hike, jump-rope, rebounder, swim, spin, boxing
- Strength/Toning – 15 minutes – machines, free weights, body-weight exercises, pilates, ball work
- Flexibility/Stretching – 10 minutes – yoga moves, stretching
- Spot-training for sculpting – can be substituted for strength/toning

To find out more about what to do to tone and strengthen the aging body, I recommend: Age-Defying Fitness by Marilyn Moffatt and Carole B. Lewis. A key benefit for the older exerciser is keeping the joints supple and the skin taut. It is critical to move, every day!

Extreme exercise does not apply here. When you have been off your Mad-Body Mountain for at least two months, and are maintaining your weight, you can move to some of these more intense programs – just be aware of the feedback from your body and do not overdo it!

The Intense Stuff

- Cross-fit
- Boot Camps
- Mud Runs
- Marathons

- Triathlons
- P90X

These are all great programs, and produce amazing results. But, if you are Stage 2 or 3, you may end up injured or in so much pain you will never go again. Wait until you have been off the mountain for a good three to four months, feel amazing and need to challenge your body.

Modifying for Injuries/Illness – if you are injured, or are recovering from a past injury, do not try to do all the movements and machines in a circuit training or weight-room – check with a qualified trainer or physical therapist to make sure you are not going to aggravate something. Areas to watch out for and protect:

- Back
- Neck
- Knee
- Hip
- Shoulder
- Wrists

Anything that was hurt or hurts! Even if it was years ago. Take care of your body and protect it.

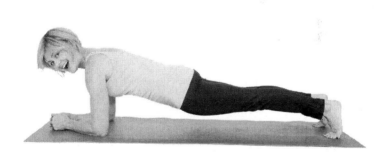

Deb's Exercise Program

At 63, I exercise less than I did in my 40s, but I exercise smarter, and I exercise every day. I know what my body responds to and how to tone-up, quickly! One of my favorite exercises to tone the core – planks! It is all about holding the pose, pulling in your stomach and just seeing how long you can stay that way. Your stomach needs to start vibrating from the effort, to get results. Then, you increase by a few seconds every time. Another is push-ups – great for increasing upper-body strength and they can be done anywhere, any time. Start with however many you can do and increase daily. When you fall off the wagon, just start over.

My other absolute daily go-to exercise – yoga and yoga-lates. I do a 10 to 15 minute session every day. I like Hatha Yoga and the Sun Salute for an overall toning that I can do quickly. Then, some Mat Pilates moves for lengthening, working abs and toning all over. You can get great arm muscles from upside-down yoga poses (downward dog with alternating lifted legs and dips into cobra, then Upward Dog to Downward Dog and repeat.) One of my favorite yoga teachers is Shiva Rea. I credit her DVDs with getting me toned for the photo shoots in this book.

As a wake-up, I like to jump on my mini-rebounder for about 5 minutes, jumping and twisting and including about 12 to 15 deep squats and jump-ups, ending with health bounces. This has totally toned my thighs and tush. Three minutes of rebounding is equivalent to jogging for ten minutes, so it is a great way to tone and energize!

I have incorporated a variety of daily "movement" to stay supple, lean and strong. It controls any of the back, knee and neck pain I used to have. If I miss a day, I hurt. If I have to sit in a car for too long, I hurt. Mitigating the effects of years in front of a computer, three rear-enders, commuting by car and now being seated for consultations, writing and webinars requires constant vigilance and daily effort.

In addition to daily yoga and exercise, I swear by twice-a-month chiropractic sessions to manage my neck, back and hip pain. Without these, I start hurting and even yoga cannot help. If you don't like chiropractic, try a good massage. The right style can work wonders! Just don't mask the pain or live on pain-killers. It is possible to reverse the damage with a naturally anti-inflammatory diet, exercise and the right lifestyle.

Now, your diet, exercise and supplements are under control. What is next? YOU! *Your Self-Care* – how you nurture and restore your soul and spirit. How you recover when another of those tough days or sad life-events occurs. How you stay away from your bad habits and off the mountain.

Step 6 – Develop Your Self-Care and Stress-Management Strategy

Developing the Self-Care Program

As a hard-working professional and parent, you often push your personal time and needs to the side. One client, a mom married to an airline pilot, refers to herself as the "married single parent". She is often left for days to run a household with a two and four-year old, plus her home-based business, plus take care of herself. She had become very run-down, largely due to the interrupted sleep cycles and trying to do her business after the children went to bed. Her body was depleted and she was dragging through the day.

Her request was for nutritional suggestions to help with the low-energy, but I was most concerned with the ongoing lack-of-sleep. You can nutrient and create energy, but sleep is precious and so restorative, that, after prolonged periods without it, your health will suffer. The key for her was to unplug from her work and day and give herself a 20-minute decompress cycle, prior to going to bed. I also put her on vitamins, minerals and some melatonin, plus some green smoothies for nutrition.

If you do not let yourself decompress prior to bed, with lowered lighting, some soft music or journaling, your mind cannot easily turn-off. You need to develop your own night-time ritual. If you are not going to bed the same time as your partner, where you can soothe each other, kiss each other goodnight and drift off to sleep, then you have to give yourself some loving care. I am up a full three to four hours past my husband, and this means my solitary ritual is essential. My ritual includes washing my face, using my Chi machine for a few minutes to loosen and relax my spine, doing some journaling or list the projects for the next day, taking my melatonin and then heading off to bed.

But, the most important ritual is one I adopted after watching the movie, "Book of Life". While somewhat banal, this animated feature talked about remembering the ancestors and how, if you are not remembered after death, you go to the "bad place". So, now I say good-night to my departed loved ones. The list is long, beginning with my son, moving through my loving dog, Boomer, and all my relatives. Even my former in-laws. I say Good-night to them all, and end with, "I love you." and "Thank you for loving me." I look up at the stars, breathe in the night air and am soothed. I used to lie awake for several minutes, all kinds of thoughts running through my mind and now, I fall asleep very quickly.

Another self-care mechanism is to let yourself cry when moved to do so. Tears are a special release of toxins and too many of us suppress them. One client came to me and told me she was having a terrible time urinating. She would get cramps and only a bit would come out. This was the client whose husband had passed six months prior, at Christmas. The doctors had tested her urine, found protein crystals that should not be there, put her through a battery of tests, and had no answer. My intuition told me it was due to the suppression of grief and not letting her tears flow. When we hold in our emotions, we create a chemical response in the body. I took her hands, looked deep into her eyes, and asked her, "Have you let yourself really grieve the loss of your husband?" She looked back at me and said, "No." I said, "It is time. Your body is telling you to let it out and cry." She began crying. I cried with her and we cried for a long time.

I sent her home with some supplements to support her system and told her to spend the next week really experiencing the loss and letting the tears flow. One week later, we were able to begin her weight-loss and health-recovery program. Her health-recovery program included joining a grief-support group at the local church. She is now a facilitator for that group, and dating a wonderful man. She is glowing with health and loves her new, sixty pounds lighter body!

If you are trying to stay strong after a loss or tragedy, don't. There will be times when you have to keep it together. But, when moved to cry, let it out. The tears themselves are washing away the toxins, releasing the memories and allowing you to heal. If you need to bawl, do it. Sometimes I look at pictures of my prior family, and think of all the happy times, and I let the tears flow. Write in a journal. Write a book. Write a blog. Call a friend. Join a grief support group. It all helps the healing process. Join us in the Facebook group: MadBody Mountain. We will help you. See Resources for how to reach us.

The best mantra I teach my clients going through something is: "This too shall pass". And, you have to get strong to grow. The best present we can give ourselves is to honor our own needs and give ourselves a thriving body that can take on anything and rebound from anything.

It is all right to give in to the sadness. It is not all right to live there and never rise up. Set up your life to stay off the mountain.

These are the foundational practices that will make the difference:

Self-care:

- Relaxation (at least 1 hour a day "unplugged": lunch with no electronics, no TV or computer one hour before bed)
- Recreation (fun stuff, not TV or Facebook!) – preferably outside
- Study/Personal Growth (read, watch videos, listen to self-help/motivational CD)
- Emotions/Stress-Management Techniques – meditation, yoga, deep breathing
- Career Satisfaction (find something you love to do that is not work, but joy)
- Work/Life Balance (Schedule in family and friend time and keep it!)
- Family (Your family is your support system – whether by birth or by creating it from friends)
- Relationship (Someone to love who loves you and helps you be who you want to be)
- Attitude and Gratitude Journal – five minutes a day jotting down what you are grateful for
- Happy Body – which needs:

Chemistry: Probiotics (keeping your body strong and healthy and absorbing nutrition); healthy liver, healthy adrenals, healthy digestion, healthy mind, healthy hormonal levels; supplements to fill in gaps

Hydration: ½ your weight in ounces of water daily

Alkalinity and controlling Insulin: get two plates of vegetables or one green juice/smoothie a day

Right amount and right kind of calories: your best eating style (paleo, vegetarian, etc.)

Exercise: 30 to 45 minutes a day of movement that your body loves and that you will do, willingly

Restorative Sleep: 7 to 8 hours a night, every night!

Develop Your
Stress-Management Strategy

Stress is attacking every cell of our body, every day. Stress depletes us as though we had just run a mile. We pant, our hearts race, we cannot catch our breath. Then, we repeat this day after day. The organs and digestion suffer. The muscles tense.

The level of support needed to address this solely from our food is totally insufficient. Our body is simply going to stay Mad and In Revolt and we will stay on Mad-Body Mountain if we cannot lessen the effects of stress on the body. Self-care such as yoga, taking walks, meditating, journaling, deep-breathing, all help. Nutrition will help you deal with stress. Essential-fatty acids found in fish, such as: salmon, tuna, herring, sardines, mackerel, and plant-based foods: grasses, nuts and seeds, all help the brain function at its best. Staying off the foods that trigger sugar-spikes will keep you thinking better. Drinking water instead of caffeine and alcohol will help you. Green juices and raw foods will help. Taking the supplements that support brain and gut will also help. These can be Omega-3s, probiotics, Gingko, plus the foundation vitamins and minerals.

Another key way to deal with stress is to exercise. Running, dancing, jump-roping, swimming, biking, hiking, walking, working out with weights. All of these will burn off the adrenaline and help the body to calm down, while pushing blood through the body, carrying nutrients and removing toxins.

Read a good book or lose yourself in a fun novel or magazine. Soak in the tub!

You can also take some creative down-time. Try learning a new language, musical instrument, painting, drawing, journaling. Just take your mind somewhere it can leave the stress behind. It will pay you back handsomely!

Friends are a huge factor is helping us handle stress. If you don't have a close friend who can listen without judging or preaching, reach out to a church support group, or a counselor. Just don't keep it bottled up inside. Stress is toxic and you need to let it go!

Ask for help. It is there for you. Don't do this alone.

Managing Emotions, Setbacks and Plateaus

It is really important to identify emotional blocks and emotional-eating triggers. Try keeping a journal to track what you were feeling when you ate something that you know is a problem for you – figure out if you eat when you are sad, angry, happy or just bored. I have pet names for these types of eating cycles: Bratty, Brainless Binger is when I am just eating and not even realizing it. Chatty, Chewy Cathy is when I am partying and chowing down while gabbing away and not realizing it. Debbie Downer is when I am depressed and eating to feel better. Mean, Midnight Muncher is when I am bored, possibly depressed, and staying up too late.

The way to handle these cycles is to realize when you are in one and stop!

I believe that the majority of us can control our urges in good emotional times. What we have to do is have coping mechanisms for the tough times. This is when we really have to call on all our tricks and tools. Here are some of the tips I have used with my clients to handle stress eating and urges:

Managing Stress-Eating and Getting Restorative Sleep

25 Tips to Handle Stress-Eating:

1. Drink Water when you think you are hungry
2. Identify Timing of Urges and Triggers
3. Journal every bite and emotions at time of eating
4. Keep hands busy
5. Chew 35 - 50X – every bite!
6. Wear something so constricting you feel it and can't put another morsel in – Seriously!
7. Move, take a walk, dance, clean, organize your closet (try outfits on)
8. Eat low-calorie, high-fiber munchies – veggies
9. Build bite-size serving portions (trail mix)
10. Call someone who will understand
11. Cook/prepare something healthy
12. Journal your thoughts and why you are bored or stressed
13. Deep breathe, moving your stomach in and out
14. Exercise – 10 minutes will help
15. Yoga
16. Play with makeup
17. Make a vision board of what you will do when you lose the

weight

18. Go To Bed Early
19. Managing Stress-Eating on the Job
20. Take a walk
21. Stretch
22. Keep healthy munchies at the desk, in your purse and briefcase
23. Journal what is going on driving your stress
24. Breathe deep and move your stomach
25. Play music

Seven Ways to De-Stress Before Trying to Sleep:

1. No electronic activity for one hour before bed
2. Dim the lights
3. Deep-breathe and really relax
4. Tighten parts of your body, starting with the feet and ankles, moving up the body, release, breathe four times deeply between the sections of your body, while in bed, with lights out – then tense the entire body, hold, breathe four times in and out – This should release a great deal of stress and help you fall asleep
5. Exercise at least 3 hours before bed, except yoga
6. No food three hours before
7. Take a melatonin supplement to generate serotonin, the "happy hormone" that helps us relax and sleep

When you have a super-stressful day, and you just cannot calm-down, there are some mantras that may help:

Mantras for Getting Through
Mad-Body Attacks

Preface: For many months after my years of strife, I had to calm my mind and provide the nourishment for my soul. I had lost my job, home, son, marriage of thirty years, my retirement savings and my desire for life. I was living alone, with no job, at fifty-one. I was so sad and tired I was not sure I would make it, or even wanted to. All that kept me going was the thought that there was someone I was meant to help that was in worse shape than me. Today, I still use these mantras and techniques when I need them. I hope they provide solace for you.

Dealing with Anxiety: Deep breathe in and out from the stomach, 6 counts in through your nose, hold for 1 count, 6 counts out through your mouth. Repeat three to five times, then say (and mean it):

"This too shall pass!"

Feeling Lacking and/or guilty for wanting more: Breathe per above and say:

"I Am Enough,

I Have Enough,

I Do Enough – but I want more, so More, Please!"

Feeling Unloved or Un-Lovely: Stand in front of a mirror, gaze lovingly at yourself, smile, take a deep breath and say

"I am Beautiful, I am Loving, I am Lovable
and I am Worthy of Love!"

Repeat three times and get stronger and louder each time, ending with your hands up over your head. Believe It!

Nourishing Yourself Mindfully: Hold the supplements, water or food in your hand, gaze down, breathe deeply and say:

"Heal My Body, Nourish My Soul, Calm My Mind."

(grow my hair, or release the fat, or give me energy – insert your choice or make one up for the fourth). Then, every time you put in another bite, or take another vitamin or drink some water or a smoothie or green juice, think that phrase to yourself. Galvanize those cells into action!

Spiritual Support

My daily spiritual practice involves connecting with a higher-being and tuning into what I need to be doing to fulfill what I believe to be my purpose in life. For many of my clients, they turn to their religion and God and it will help them tremendously. I support whatever process and belief system gives you solace and strength. Call on your own personal guide/god/universal manager and bring peace and serenity to your being. It will help you get off the mountain.

Chapter 6 –
Make Your Relationships
Work for You

Getting sexy, lean and strong is not just about the physical person you are helping to heal and emerge. It is about your personal self, your emotions, goals and dreams. If you are in a relationship that creates pain and doubt, you have to decide if you can recover or you need to remove yourself. If the person who you spend your energy on is not trying to improve and reach another level, why would you stay there? Relationships are a two-way street. If you are missing something then you may find yourself filling the hole with food.

Instead of shoving in that brownie or handful of chips, try telling yourself what Aibileen taught to her charge, Mae Mobley, in "The Help": "You is kind, you is smart, you is impo'tant" Or, in my words: "You are Beautiful, you are Loving, you are Lovable and you are Worthy of Love!"

Believe it and then take steps to take care of the beautiful body, mind and heart you have. Do not let anyone trample on it and do not allow yourself to end up stuck on Mad Body Mountain.

Step 7 –
Make Your Relationships
Work for You

Many times you may be dealing with lack of support from your spouse or significant other, or family member(s). You have to get them on your side by explaining where you are on the mountain and why you need to come down, and ask for their support. If they just won't give it, you have to tell them this is what you have to do, and you will do it no matter what! It is no longer an option to submit to their choice of bad food or lack of exercise in order to keep the relationship intact. This relationship is now toxic. You either have to heal it or drop it. If you cannot do either, it will be almost impossible to come down off your mountain. If you don't want to divorce your mate or family, you have to learn to stand your ground at home and in social situations.

If your family members and friends cannot support you through the process of cleaning up your eating and habits to support your body's needs, it is going to be difficult to stay on-track. I encourage you to seek out someone who can help support you through the process – a health coach or life coach or just a good, healthy friend. The benefits of getting off the mountain are worth having to push-back on a family member who thinks "you should be able to have one cookie, bite of cake, some ice cream – It isn't going to kill you!" But, over the long haul, it actually will. Until you are off the Mad-Body Mountain and can handle the little amount of cheating, don't give in!!!

Now you have gone through the self-analysis, determined where you are on the mountain, asked yourself what factors you grew up with and how you can break-off from the bad habits. Here is where the family has to get connected with your goals and bless them, if they cannot understand and accept them.

Getting to the bottom of the mountain can be hard when the people you live with or hang-out with don't want to come down with you. It will take too much energy to convert them to your plan, so you are going to have to go it alone, with some new buddies that you select and recruit to your side.

Just know that you will get down. You will turn your health around and you are going to be exactly who you want to be! You are going to have to address all the factors, and one of those is your love relationship. If there are problems, these have to be addressed to achieve your optimal health and wellness.

Fixing the Problems
in a Love Relationship

One day the pain of whatever you are forcing yourself to tolerate becomes too great and, in addition to all the new food and lifestyle habits, you must rid yourself of the emotional baggage. You cannot fully heal and achieve optimal health when you are shackled by the terrible emotional toll a bad relationship, work or home environment creates. You have to break free of these bonds as well! This means either leaving or tackling the problems head-on.

After slogging through twelve years of a volatile, extremely wearing relationship with my new husband, I discovered two amazing books that taught me a lot about why we were so dysfunctional. We read them together and worked through the exercises. We were able to get to a place where we could actually communicate and not set each other off, and learned to quickly mend the relationship when things got too heated.

I love these books and tell all my clients who have communication issues with their significant others about them. The first was The Five Love Languages, by Gary Chapman. The second was the book, Wired for Love by Dr. Stan Tatkin. Using books like these can really help, if both partners are committed to working things out.

The key teaching in Wired for Love is that we are one of three styles of people, based on how we were loved or not as children: wave, anchor or island. As a couple, we have to create a "couple-bubble" and put the other as the most important priority in our life. We must protect and nurture each other, not tear each other down. To do that, we need to know the other person and what they will need when feeling upset or let-down. We commit to be their source of support and to soothe the angry beast.

This seems simple and, for some couples, it is. For my first husband and I it was, but he was actually more in-tune and careful of my feelings than I was of his. I was the insensitive wave who bowled people over and he was the anchor, holding it all together.

According to Dr. Tatkin, anchors are the people who were loved and had a great childhood so they are very secure and attuned to other's needs. Then there are the waves, which is me, and the islands, which is my second husband. We faced challenges as a couple as we both had difficult childhoods and this created insecurities and inabilities to express ourselves without upsetting each other. I become a "tsunami-wave" and he becomes a "volcano-island" when we feel threatened, attacked, overlooked or belittled, even if that is not what the other intended. It used to take hours, even days and weeks, to patch things up between us. One small comment, taken the wrong way, could turn into a huge blow-up.

What Dr. Tatkin teaches us to do is learn to overlook the tone or the implied anger and wait for the storms to subside, then approach the other in the recommended way to soothe the situation. If the relationship is worth keeping, then you may have to do some changing. I had to learn how to not take everything my new husband said so personally. He had to learn that I am very sensitive to teasing and do not handle it well. We both had to learn how to not push each other's buttons. Our conversations and discussions are no longer at-risk of degenerating into shouting matches, each vying for the win. I come to the relationship understanding him better, and he me.

Here are some of the behaviors we have agreed to embrace. We have morning and evening rituals so each feels seen and loved. We make time for each other to share things during the day. We set time aside for just us.

Some of the exercises from Wired for Love that you may need to do:

- Negotiate a new relationship contract
- Find ways to stay in communication
- Don't let problems fester
- Learn how to explain what you want without having to yell or be argumentative
- Find a way to cool-down before tackling the tough conversations

I have turned many of my clients struggling with their partners onto these books and have seen some great results. They may help you as well!

Chapter 7 – Time to Hike Down!

Step 8 – Strap On Your Pack and Let's Get Down!

Now is the time to final-check your plan. You have designed a plan that is tailored to you and your needs. It meets your lifestyle and allows you to fit the right choices in, daily. You have figured out which foods your body loves and will perform best on. You got through Strengthen, Repair and Prepare and feel ready to do more. You developed an exercise plan that will work for you and you are dealing with emotions, stress and your relationships. Now, you can put all these tools in your back-pack, pick up your hiking stick and Get Off That Mountain!

For some, the first few weeks after Strengthen, Repair and Prepare are all about the quick results – if you need to drop weight in a week, you can do a cleanse. If you are toxic, do a mini-fast. If you just want to slowly drop pounds, begin with dropping all the junk, add in super-nutritious food every day, get in the exercise, and keep this up for at least thirty-three days. Make sure you have the right supplements to support you as they will help you keep up the exercise, sleep enough and drop the weight.

Just remember, this is the break-in period – depending on where you are starting from, you may be journeying down for 30, 45, 70, 90 days or more. No matter how long it takes, you will have developed habits that will take you back to Sexy, Lean and Strong as long as you keep them up. Every day you will need to be mindful of your choices. You know how to make the right ones, so, when you cheat or back-slide, you can fix it. Just don't let yourself cheat too much. You must get in your daily exercise and self-care. If a critical relationship is rocky, you have to build-in time to address that. It is all worth it, but it all needs to be handled. Too many times at our later age in life, we make excuses for not tackling the tough stuff, whether the relationship dynamic or our cravings. They both have to be handled. No more saying, "I will worry about this tomorrow, next month or next year." No more fooling yourself that you can take the weight off in a month or so. You are not going to do that. That is why you are on that mountain!

If you are dealing with loss, then now is the time to make sure you have a support network in place – either a counselor, grief support group, church group, or just great friends. Do not attempt to get through your descent alone!

Can You Cheat?

There will be days where you just have to cheat! That is OK, sort-of. My advice is you can cheat at Stage 1 a big 10% of the time. At Stage 2, 8% and at Stage 3, no more than 5%. Think about how many good meals and snacks it will take to get to your goal. If you are eating five times a day, then, over 90 days that is 450 meals/snacks. If you eat less than stellar for 45, that is a lot for the body to handle. It can only do it when you are balanced, getting enough nutrition the rest of the time and take the time to work it off. Take a look at the exercise/calories burned chart in the Appendix. I tell my clients, if you want to eat that bread, cake, cookie, ice cream or drink that wine, you better be ready to exercise it away within twelve hours!

Trail Markers: Weight Versus Inches

Most folks feel they are failing if the pounds do not decrease. They will weigh themselves every day, frustrated when the scale creeps up. First, I advise you to weigh twice a week, first thing Monday morning and again on Friday night. Weight can fluctuate daily. The movement during the week is what is important.

If you are exercising and eating right, often the weight can stay the same but you can actually be tightening up, building muscle and actually getting smaller. This is why my focus is on getting lean and strong, not skinny. There are some key measurements to watch during your climb down. Collect these measurements at the beginning of the program, again every ten days or so, and when you reach the Valley. A good sign is a shrinking belly, waist and hips, with growing biceps and forearms. When this happens, the weight is often the same and sometimes, more. Don't be afraid to put on some pounds if you are shrinking at the same time! If the arm muscles or thigh muscles increase, and the belly and waist decreases, but the pounds are the same, it is still cause to celebrate! Muscle is denser than fat, burns more calories per pound and getting smaller is getting smaller. The weight-loss may take more time, but it will happen. It is all about how your body releases fat and what causes it to hold onto the fat. Now that you know which foods make it happy and lean, just eat more of them, and less of the bad ones!

Key Measurements:

- Neck
- Wrist
- Forearm
- Bicep
- Bust/Chest
- Belly-button
- Hips
- Upper Thigh
- Calf

Two important measurements you must care about are the belly and the waist. If you are a man and your belly is more than 39", you are at risk for heart-disease. If you are a woman and it is over 35", you are at risk for heart-disease. There is no fudging this, and you have to take it seriously. If you are over those measurements, you are probably a high Stage 2 or 3. You need to deal with this, and now! Just ask yourself, do you want to dance at your child's wedding or hold your grandchildren?

Managing Plateaus

Let's assume you have been journeying down the mountain for 90 days. You may have hit a plateau. You are getting bored with the same foods. You are tired of going to the gym. The scale is stuck at a certain spot. You are ready to throw in the towel. Nothing is working! Sit down and look at what you are really doing. Make sure you have kept track of what you are eating, and when. You may have missed some snack-cycles, but you are working out more. Guess what? You need to eat more! Add in some protein, especially if you are developing muscles. Eat every two to three hours, just a bite even. You need to make sure your body does not feel "starved" due to wanting more calories. You are a finely-tuned machine and, you can go out-of-balance easily. It is up to you to make sure you are eating enough to keep all the cells satisfied and releasing fat. You may have to cut back on whatever starches you snuck back in. Be honest! Plateaus happen because either the body is tired, bored, hungry, upset emotionally, or unexercised. Stay on those supplements! They will help you fill in the gaps.

Dealing With Temptation
At Special Events

You have a special occasion coming up – family reunion, wedding, graduation, cruise. You have done really well. Why not slack-off?

When you have been good for 90 days straight, lost at least 20 pounds or more, feel great, look great, it is super-easy to tell yourself, "Just one bite, taste, slice." *Time to refocus!*

What is the ultimate goal here? When you look at the tempting food, what are you saying to yourself? Try this: "I eat to nourish my body and mind. I eat to rebuild my cells and recraft my body. I move and run and dance and work-out to create the best body I can. I love my body and it loves me and I love how I feel when I eat the best way for my body and my health." Then, decide if you really want that morsel!

Now, say you are going to an event and you know there will be all kinds of tempting, not-so-good-for you foods. What do you do to stave off these tempting goodies? Here are my tricks for making sure my clients and I stay on-track:

- Exercise the day of the party and the day after
- Eat healthfully before the party to fill up on something good
- Drink a glass of water before any alcoholic drink, and after
- Eat your veggies first, then the protein and then a starch; and trade bread for dessert or starch – you cannot have all three at one sitting

84

- Go light on dairy products
- Try a bit of everything but do not gorge on any one item
- Stop when you are satisfied, not full

When you are going to be at a special event and there will be lots of goodies, I actually tell my clients to let the Sexy, Lean and Strong plan go for that day, as long as they commit to cleaning up their act the very next day. You cannot cheat multiple days in a row and maintain the weight loss. After you reach the valley, you can cheat one day a month and it will not do much damage. If you do go off-track, my rule is never get more than four pounds over or under your ideal weight. This keeps you in-check and it is easy to get back to the ideal weight in just a few days.

When we cheat, we are heaping more work on our livers and other organs and we have to reverse it. That is where your favorite cleanse and mini-fast comes in. The whole concept of how many calories is not as critical as what those calories are made up of. If they are nutrient-dense, less will fill you up and sustain you longer. So, after a binge-day, the next day or two will need to consist of eating salads and green smoothies or veggie stir-frys with a bit of lean protein, or, soups and juicing.

I love the recipes in *The Liver Cleanse* by Dr. Sandra Cabot for main dishes, soups and smoothies and in *Essential Green Smoothies*, by Madeline Eyer. These recipes taste great and are super-nutritious. Eating from these books will make your body feel marvelous and get you back to normal, fast.

Again, it is all a work-in-progress. Getting off the mountain can take weeks, months or even years. Be patient! Love yourself all the way through the descent.

Chapter 8 – Staying on the Path – No Matter What!

While you are coming down the mountain, you are going to run into obstacles. It is up to you to get over them, around them or go through them. Avoiding them is no longer an option. This is one of the reasons you are on the mountain in the first place!

Step 9: Stay On the Path – Adjust As Needed

Wrong People – Either leave or figure out how to change the dynamic to support your health – physical, spiritual and mental

Wrong Place – If you are finding that, everywhere you turn, someone is beating you down for your ideas, maybe it is time to move! No matter how old you are, you are allowed to thrive and not just survive!

Wrong Mind-set – When you are attacked or teased for wanting to eat better, exercise more, not watch so much TV, you start succumbing to fit-in. Don't!!! You can control your mind and what you do. Letting others take control will only put you back on the Mad-Body Mountain!

Wrong Focus – Stop worrying about what size you were ten or fifteen years ago. Embrace the healthy you you are creating. Love you, who you are today and what you will become. Focus on the good and not the bad. Praise your eyes, laugh, love and caring for others.

Wrong Foods – You know what they are by now – sugar, flour, white foods, over-processed foods, non-organic and chemically-altered, toxins – alcohol, pesticides, and any foods that your body does not really love.

To get to the valley, you should have a mental checklist that reads like this:

Schedule, schedule, schedule – shopping, cooking, packing snacks and meals, exercise, self-care

Strategies:

- Getting your family and friends to support you – or -
- Doing it without any immediate-family support
- Church, on-line community or local meet-up for help
- Tracking and adjusting the plan when you hit a plateau
- Metabolism slow-down and Busting Plateaus Strategies
- Trying new diets/eating programs
- Trying new exercise programs and activities
- Quickie-Meals and Snacks to Keep You Energized
- Family Outings/Holidays – what is your plan to handle them?
- Friends and their events – how will you stay on-track?
- Cravings and emotional hard-times – what are your coping mechanisms?

Daily Practice – Attitude and Gratitude:

- The Mindset – Mindful choices consistently made yield optimal health
- Daily Mantras and Self-Programming for Success
- Mindful choices every day – not just food--who you allow to influence how you feel, what you say to yourself, how you get over disappointment or back-sliding
- Mind over matter – over cravings, sadness, anger
- What to do when you slip-up
- Creating your "Happiness Corner" in your mind

Just as I have overcome everything thrown at me – so can you. It will take planning and commitment, but the rewards are worth it. Every day you have to be mindful of who you are, what you want and how to create it and maintain it. Every day you have to choose not to self-sabotage or postpone the healthy path. I know you can do this because I and so many others have done it. How someone is or is not treating you is no excuse for letting it hurt your body by making bad choices. Join me in Sexy, Lean and Strong Valley!

Chapter 9 – Live in Sexy, Lean and Strong Valley, Forever!

Step 10: Celebrate Your Arrival In Sexy, Lean And Strong Valley!

Now, Celebrate Your Descent!

You Did It!!! You have lost the weight, have a daily practice of caring for your body, and you manage stress effectively and naturally. If you were on medication, your doctor has probably reduced or eliminated it.

This does not mean now you can go back to eating all the junk-y, fun foods or even the healthy foods your body does not like. This means you embrace the new you, cherish your healthy and lean body, and treat it like a precious jewel, one that can tarnish or be damaged easily. You accept that there is a new way to live, one that energizes your body's cells, gives them what they need, and that will keep you off medication and thriving! Eat clean, think clean, live clean and grow healthier every day!

Living in Sexy, Lean and Strong Valley requires total mindfulness and commitment for the rest of your life. But, it will be easy now as you will have spent the past 90 days or more developing this skill and the right habits. You give yourself non-food rewards – special treats like massages, facials, manicures and pedicures, movies, trips, clothes. (You will need lots of new clothes when you come off Mad-Body Mountain!)

Another way to celebrate is to help others trapped on their own Mad-Body Mountain. You can share some of the tips in this book, or others you discover. Your favorite recipes or exercise program. Your favorite night-time calming rituals.

I make it a point to be informed of the new findings in fitness and nutrition. Even though one would think that there cannot be much new left to discover, new twists and approaches are found all the time. Keep tuned-in and you will find new ways to stay committed to staying off Mad-Body Mountain.

If you are beginning your descent, please write and let me know. We want to support you on your journey and celebrate when you arrive at your goal! If you have questions, I will be happy to give you my input.

To the New, Sexy, Lean and Strong You!!!

Deb Dutcher, Health Coach

www.energyunlimitedcoach.com and www.sexyleanandstrong.com

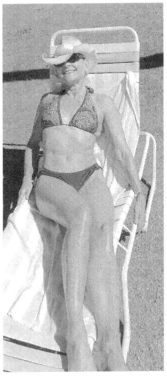

The End Result – Sexy, Lean and Strong at 62!

Acknowledgements

To Tom, my long-suffering Island-man from your Tsunami-wave woman. You are my rock and I could not have done this without your support.

To my clients, who taught me so much about the body's ability to recover, and especially those who allowed me to share their journey.

To my family, your love means everything.

To my friends, who saw me through it all: divorce, losing my son to drugs, rejection by my daughter, losing my ranch, retirement savings and livelihood, then the challenges of a second marriage. You have all helped me to become the thriving woman I am today.

To my teachers, mentors and coaches. I never stop learning and you never stop teaching and supporting!

To my daughter, Raquele. You have become a lovely woman and I love and cherish you.

To my son, Abraham, the boy with the Golden Heart who never got to show the world all you could be. I miss you every day and I do what I do in your name.

To the dynamic team from Klein Graphics, Randy and Christina Klein, for all the beautiful art for the cover and the illustrations.

And finally, to Dr. Myron Wentz, who created the wonderfully-effective nutritional products that helped me get off *my* Mad-Body Mountain, and has helped hundreds of thousands recover their health. This book celebrates the journey down Mad-Body Mountain to Sexy, Lean and Strong -- after 50!

About the Author

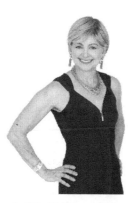

A former high-tech VP, Deb went through a divorce, death of her son, losing her health, home and retirement, to become a thriving, sexy, lean and strong gal who, at 63, has the energy and drive to accomplish anything. She has helped thousands to turn their health around and get down Mad-Body Mountain, teaching them how to take themselves on and win.

Deb runs a private Health Coaching and Corporate Wellness Consulting practice in Brentwood, California – Energy Unlimited Coach. She is a Featured Expert Writer for "Wealthy Woman" e-magazine, and an international speaker. Deb is a Certified Integrative Health Coach through the Institute for Integrative Nutrition and a Certified Nutrition Advisor for Sanoviv Medical Institute.

Deb founded Abe's Heart of Gold Foundation to reach-out to youth-at-risk in memory of her son, Abraham Linder. Her goal is to teach these youths how to manage their anger and depression and use nutrition and a healthy lifestyle to overcome, instead of deadening their pain with drugs and alcohol.

All proceeds from this book will be used to support this effort.

Contacts and Resources

Author:

deb@energyunlimited.biz
www.facebook.com/deb.dutcher
www.SexyLeanandStrong.com
www.facebook.com/sexyleanandstrong
www.facebook.com/groups/madbodymountain
www.energyunlimitedcoach.com
www.abesheartofgold.org

Resources:

Trusted Supplement Providers:
www.usana.com (Vitamins, supplements and weight-loss programs)
www.products.mercola.com – (Vitamins and supplements)
www.weilvitaminadvisor.com – (Vitamins and supplements)
www.womenshealthnetwork.com – (Vitamins and supplements)

References

Books:

Cabot, Sandra. The Liver Cleansing Diet (SBC International, 2013)

Chapman, Gary. The Five Love Languages (Northfield Publishing, 2004)

Eyer, Madeline. Essential Smoothies (Heartlight, 2013)

Kalina, Laura. Low-Glycemic Meals in Minutes (True Health Global Publishing, 2007, 2014)

MacWilliam, Lyle. Nutrisearch Comparative Guide to Nutritional Supplements. (Northern Dimensions Publishing, 2007)

Moffat, Marilyn. Age-Defying Fitness (Peachtree Publishers, 2006)

Pert, Candice. Molecules of Emotion (Scribner, 1997)

Rosenthal, Joshua. Integrative Nutrition. New York (Integrative Nutrition Publishing, 2007).

Santillo, Humbart. Food Enzymes, The Missing Link to Radiant Health (Hohm Press, 1993)

Tatkin, Stan. Wired for Love (New Harbinger Publications, Inc., 2011)

Wentz, Myron. Invisible Miracles –- The Revolution in Cellular Nutrition (Medicis, S.C., 2002)

Appendices

Appendix I - Dietary Programs

Note: There are over one hundred dietary programs, and more popping up every day. I use a few key programs when developing plans for clients. I am going to summarize them here. To me it is more important to eat the foods that make your body happy and healthy than worry about what to label that style of eating. I like to eat a blend of Paleo/Low-glycemic with some dairy and grain every now and then. Plus dark chocolate!

- Gluten-free – Eating only gluten-free foods
- Low-Glycemic – Eating low-glycemic foods that do not spike blood sugar, staying under 55 on the Glycemic Index; eating protein and fiber at every meal and snack
- Paleo – Removing grain, sugar and dairy from the diet; eating grass-fed animal protein, organic poultry, wild-caught fish, organ meats, vegetables, nuts, seeds, honey, maple syrup, oats, butter, coconut oil
- Raw foods – Eating only raw vegetables, fruit, nuts, seeds and fats. Nothing cooked
- Vegetarian – No animal protein, including fish or dairy.

Appendix II - Exercise/Activity Chart and Calories Burned

Activity & Calories Burned per Hour – Based on Body Weight of 155 lbs

Aerobics, general	457
Aerobics, high impact	493
Backpacking, Hiking with pack	493
Ballroom dancing, fast	387
Basketball game, competitive	563
Bowling	211
Boxing, sparring	633
Calisthenics, light, pushups, situps	246
Calisthenics, fast, pushups, situps	563
Carrying 16 to 24 lbs, upstairs	422
Carrying 25 to 49 lbs, upstairs	563
Circuit training, minimal rest	563
Cleaning, dusting	176
Cross country snow skiing, slow	493
Cross country skiing, racing	985
Cycling, <10mph, leisure bicycling	281
Cycling, >20mph, racing	1126
Cycling, 10-11.9mph, light	426
Gardening, general	281
General cleaning	246
Golf, driving range	211
Golf, general	317
Gymnastics	281
Health club exercise	387
Hiking, cross country	422
Horesback riding, saddling horse	246
Housework, light	176
Housework, moderate	246
Ice skating, < 9 mph	387
Ice skating, rapidly	633

Jazzercise	422
Judo, karate, jujitsu, martial arts	704
Jumping rope, fast	844
Kayaking	352
Kick boxing	704
Loading, unloading car	211
Masseur, masseuse, standing	281
Mild stretching	176
Nursing, patient care	211
Pushing stroller, walking	176
Race walking	176
Raking lawn	303
Riding motorcycle	176
Roller blading, in-line skating	844
Roller skating	93
Rowing machine, light	246
Rowing machine, moderate	493
Rowing machine, vigorous	598
Running, 5 mph (12 minute mile)	563
Running, 6 mph (10 min mile)	704
Sit, playing with animals, light	176
Sitting, light office work	106
Skateboarding	352
Skiing, water skiing	422
Snorkeling	352
Snow shoeing	563
Snow skiing, downhill skiing, light	352
Stair machine	633
Standing, bartending, store clerk	162
Standing, playing with children, light	197
Stationary cycling, light	387
Stationary cycling, moderate	493
Stationary cycling, very vigorous	880
Stretching, hatha yoga	281
Surfing, body surfing or board surfing	211

Swimming backstroke	493
Swimming breaststroke	704
Swimming leisurely, not laps	422
Swimming sidestroke	563
Table tennis, ping pong	281
Tae kwan do, martial arts	704
Tai chi	281
Tennis playing	493
Tennis, doubles	422
Tennis, singles	563
Trampoline	246
Typing, computer data entry	106
Volleyball playing	211
Volleyball, beach	563
Walk / run, playing, moderate	281
Walk / run, playing, vigorous	352
Walking 2.0 mph, slow	176
Walking 3.5 mph, brisk pace	267
Walking downstairs	211
Walking the dog	211
Walking, pushing a wheelchair	281
Water aerobics	281
Water jogging	563
Weeding, cultivating garden	317
Weight lifting, body building, vigorous	422
Weight lifting, light workout	211

Made in the USA
San Bernardino, CA
21 March 2016